ETHICAL PROBLEMS IN DIALYSIS AND TRANSPLANTATION

DEVELOPMENTS IN NEPHROLOGY

Volume 33

The Titles published in this series are listed at the end of this volume.

Ethical problems in dialysis and transplantation

edited by

CARL M. KJELLSTRAND

Professor of Medicine, Faculty of Medicine, University of Alberta, Edmonton, Canada

and

JOHN B. DOSSETOR

Professor of Medicine, Director, Division of Bioethics, Faculty of Medicine, University of Alberta, Edmonton, Canada

KLUWER ACADEMIC PUBLISHERS
DORDRECHT / BOSTON / LONDON

Library of Congress Cataloging-in-Publication Data

Ethical problems in dialysis and transplantation / edited by Carl M.
  Kjellstrand and John B. Dossetor.
      p.   cm. -- (Developments in nephrology ; v. 33)

    ISBN 0-7923-1625-8 (HB : alk. paper)
    1. Chronic renal failure--Treatment--Moral and ethical aspects.
  2. Hemodialysis--Moral and ethical aspects. 3. Kidneys-
  -Transplantation--Moral and ethical aspects.   I. Kjellstrand, Carl
  M., 1936-   . II. Dossetor, John B. III. Series: Developments in
  nephrology ; 33.
    [DNLM: 1. Dialysis. 2. Ethics, Medical. 3. Kidney
  Transplantation.   W1 DE998ED v.33]
  RC918.R4E74 1992
  174'.25--dc20
  DNLM/DLC
  for Library of Congress   92-2962
  ISBN 0-7923-1625-8

Published by Kluwer Academic Publishers,
P.O. Box 17, 3300 AA Dordrecht, The Netherlands.

Kluwer Academic Publishers incorporates
the publishing programmes of
D. Reidel, Martinus Nijhoff, Dr W. Junk and MTP Press.

Sold and distributed in the U.S.A. and Canada
by Kluwer Academic Publishers,
101 Philip Drive, Norwell, MA 02061, U.S.A.

In all other countries, sold and distributed
by Kluwer Academic Publishers Group,
P.O. Box 322, 3300 AH Dordrecht, The Netherlands.

Printed on acid-free paper

We dedicate this book to the late E. Garner King, M.D., FRCP, FACP, our Departmental Chairman, in gratitude for enabling us to meet, and for giving us time and wherewithal to complete this book. He, better than anyone else, was able to set the stage for our academic discussions and to guide these discussions towards agreement.

We judge men by their actions,
we judge actions by their results
and from the actions
do we infer the intention.

S. Johnson

Table of contents

List of contributors

K. Atsumi, Institute for Medical Electronics, University of Tokyo, Tokyo, Japan

R. S. Barsoum, Al-Salam Hospital, Mohandessen, Cairo, Egypt

L. R. Churchill, Medical School, Chapel Hill, North Carolina, USA

R. Cranford, Department of Neurology, Hennepin County Medical Center, Minneapolis, Minnesota, USA

J. B. Dossetor, Division of Bioethics, University of Alberta, Edmonton, Canada

H. T. Engelhardt Jr., Center for Medicine and Ethics, Baylor College of Medicine, Houston, Texas, USA

A. R. Hull, The University of Texas Southwestern Medical Center at Dallas; Dallas, Texas, USA

M. Kaye, Division of Nephrology, Montreal General Hospital, Montreal, Quebec, Canada

C. M. Kjellstrand, Department of Medicine, Division of Nephrology, University of Alberta Medical School, Edmonton, Canada

M. K. Mani, Department of Nephrology, Appollo Hospital, Madras, India

V. Manickavel, Division of Bioethics, University of Alberta, Edmonton, Canada

Ren-Zong Qiu, Institute of Philosophy, Chinese Academy of Social Sciences, Beijing, China

K. D. Reddy, Department of Renal Transplantation, The Guest Hospital, Kilpuuk, Madras, India

J. R. Richards, Department of Philosophy, The Open University, Milton Keynes, United Kingdom

A. Válek, Department of Internal Medicine, Charles University Medical School, Strahoff, Prague, Czechoslovakia

A. J. Wing, United Medical & Dental School of Guy's and St. Thomas' Hospitals, London, United Kingdom

Introduction – Dialyzers and transplanters are the bioethical pointmen of modern medicine

CARL M. KJELLSTRAND & JOHN B. DOSSETOR

Chronic dialysis and renal transplantation is one of the great success stories of applied medical technology. Since the introduction and rapid dissemination of dialysis in the early 1960's, and renal transplantation a decade or so later, probably over one million patients have enjoyed years of extended life. The technology quickly spread from industrialized advanced countries in the West so that now almost every country in the world has several patients on chronic dialysis and several patients who have had renal transplantation. Clinical knowledge has rapidly advanced, early high mortality rate has fallen and survival is now counted in decades. Older patients and patients with many other diseases now benefit from these very successful treatments for chronic renal failure (ESRD).

Graphs of annual acceptance rates for dialysis show two characteristics. First, they are steadily rising without any levelling in sight, suggesting an un-met demand even in countries like Japan and USA who accept twice as many patients annually as the runner-up countries in Western Europe and Canada. Secondly, there are great differences in acceptance rates of neighbouring countries. Canada accepts less than half as many patients annually as the United States, and England and Ireland accept half as many patients as France and Italy. Criteria other than purely medical ones are obviously operating here.

Dialysis and transplantation impose ethical obligations on the physicians who practice these modes of treatment. Everywhere people are confronted with such questions as:

i) Even though everyone rations and selects, does that make such selection just?
ii) What are the ethical implications to physicians of participation in discontinuation of treatment (e.g. dialysis) when death of the patient is the inevitable consequence?
iii) As dialysis acceptance rates surge away from transplantation rates, what are the ethical implications for physicians as the market for commerce in human kidneys which is growing in many parts of the world?

These technologies cut across geographical, cultural and religious barriers. Acceptance rates for dialysis in Japan, which is a Buddhist-Shintoist country, are most similar to those of the United States, while the acceptance rates in Saudi

XV

C. M. Kjellstrand and J. B. Dossetor (eds): Ethical Problems in Dialysis and Transplantation, xv – xx.

Arabia are more similar to the Scandinavian countries than to any of the Muslim countries around it. Technology is posing the same ethical questions to the Buddhist, Hindu, Christian, Muslim and Jew. Nephrologists are stewing in a seething cauldron of ethical issues, stoked by technology – not religion, geography or other cultural influences.

One reaction to this situation is to deny that ethical tension exists. Like Dr. Pendergast in Voltaire's 'Candide' there has been a tendency to blandly state that 'this is the best of worlds' and the solutions taking place are 'the best of all'. Phrases such as 'in our country, all patients who could benefit from treatment are treated', are singularly inappropriate in the face of the wide range of national acceptance rates. Universal absolute banning of all commerce in transplant organs is the knee-jerk reaction of nearly everyone in the West but more deliberate reflection leads others to question the universal applicability of such absolutist claims. Deaths from stopping treatment masquerade as being due to diabetes or 'social cause' or 'uremia', cloaking more subtle causal factors.

In this book we have tried to lay these issues before the reader and to shed some light on how we should think about them. Is the USA accepting too many patients for dialysis and transplantation, or Canada too few? Should Saudi Arabia match Sweden in dialysis rates? Is it the role of a physician to be an advocate for individual patients or administer a rationing scheme for many? If the latter, is the rationing scheme openly and honestly revealed to the citizens who pay for it? In difficult moral questions, the farmer will give as good an answer as the professor of philosophy, said Socrates. Abandoning life by discontinuation of dialysis appears to be homicide to some, and a courageous deliverance from suffering to others. What do the religions say about this? Can one analyze it in a thoughtful, philosophical way and derive meaning?

We have asked our contributors for both the bird's eye overview and the view from the trenches, because one view is not more 'right' or 'true' than the other. Thus, the planners professional vantage point is contrasted with the view of those who struggle with insufficient resources using courage and love under brutal pressure from political or economic forces. There are the views of agnostics, Buddhists, Hindus, Muslims, Jews and Christians. We have solicited opinions from those who operate in communist, socialist and capitalist countries; there are views from ten countries and four continents. We need global discussion and a reasoned approached to ethical dilemmas spawned by a technology that has swept the globe. The number of physicians throughout the world who practice dialysis and renal transplantation is small. We gather an international meetings and discuss these ethical issues, hence the need for, and the value of, a global perspective.

The book is divided into four sections. The first section deals with those principles which are needed to analyze these dilemmas. Tristram Engelhardt confronts us with the practical questions of justice in rationing, the ethics of commercialization and the ethics of discontinuation of life support. We asked him to set down a system of secular ethics which could be used for issue analysis both in poorest

Africa and in richest Japan or America, both for atheist communism and devout Islam. We believe he has succeeded well. He gives us a system which rests on three principles: requirement for individual authorization, limited protection and limited solidarity. From these, he derives ten rules of thumb for interactions between 'moral strangers', in the field of healthcare. This system deserves our deep consideration. It recognizes the radical difference between a general secular ethics of moral strangers and the more 'content-ful' set of principles shared by 'moral friends' within, say, a community with a shared religious view of the world.

Churchill, in his chapter on Justice, somewhat surprisingly warns against ethical theories. He challenges the 'view of ethics that makes theory the final arbiter of moral problems ... the contest of 'isms' at a remove from the actual experiences of doctors, patients and families'. To the disappointment perhaps of those looking for a bridge to span the gulf between justice towards *the many* and beneficence towards the *single patient*, he warns that 'the axioms of ethics theories [used] in a deduction problem-solving process ... reflect an enfeebled moral psychology'. Each of us, according to Aristotle, is a particular 'moral craftsman', not 'assembly line conduits for cookie cutter answers'. Each group of moral actors puts a unique stamp on their decisions, just at 'pots belong to the potter or sutures to the surgeon'. Theories do not solve problems, people do, and solutions should be 'reflective oscillations between theory and practice'. With these caveats he proceeds to discuss Justice systems based on Rawlsian egalitarianism, or utilitarianism, or libertarianism (such as that of Robert Nozick) based on fundamental right. The latter is most compatible with capitalism. Nozick asks 'Why not similarly hold that some persons have to bear some costs that benefit other persons, more for the sake of the overall good?' Somewhat astonishingly, a similar point is made forcibly by Professor Ren-Zong Qiu, later, writing from communist China!

The second section addresses the intertwined issues of commercialization and modes of selection for treatment. With selection, elements of politics and power influence how medicine operates in many communities. In general, men have been 'preferred' as patients for treatment before women, the rich are favoured over the poor, and even in the most supposedly 'egalitarian' systems power leaps to the fore. Later in the book, Barsoum laments that this is obvious in selection criteria in Egypt, but these forces operate widely. We believe this issue should be clearly out on the table. Would the open and logical approach, as advocated by Barsoum, solve this problem? We hope this is true, although a view of the history of mankind perhaps makes one pessimistic.

Janet Ratcliffe Richards then logically dissects the question of commerce in kidneys. The concern here is that the destitute, who have only their own body parts left to sell, are being victimized and exploited by the rich. This has met with so much revulsion that laws against the practice have been passed, virtually without opposition, in many countries. However, she concludes, similarly to Tristram Englehardt, that there can be no absolute moral reason to prohibit the right to sell body parts between moral strangers, only of its abuse by ruthless entrepreneurs. She sees our legislation as possibly acting not so much to protect the destitute as to remove an offence to the sensibilities of those who have both money and functioning kidneys. In the next chapter a transplanter who has struggled with these problems at close range reluctantly comes to a similar conclusion.

In Hull's chapter one encounters high praise for capitalism, and in particular its success with dialysis and transplantation. In the United States, 'for-profit' dialysis is seen as a draught in which overt capitalism is blended with a hearty splash of socialized medicine (the US Government pays for this treatment) to form a potion for success which leaves other concoctions on the shelf. Compared to the US there is simply no runner-up country when it comes to treating many patients by dialysis. Finally in this section, there is a warning against creeping commercialism by the companies manufacturing medical devices and pharmaceuticals. These companies subtly mould physicians' attitudes through conditioned response rewards obtained by travel, through dinners, and gifts of equipment and 'grants'. When it seems as innocent as a handshake, how does one know when one is prostituting one's skills?

In some countries stopping dialysis has become a leading cause of death. Viewed globally, startling differences exist. In the West, discontinuation of dialysis treatment is directly related to patient age; in Japan it is inversely related to the same parameter. What does this say about our cultures and how we view and treat each other? Obviously, religious views will be paramount here, and Michael Kaye reviews how Islam, Judaism and Christianity view this problem. In the USA, as in no other country, hospitals and physicians have abrogated responsibility for solving this problem to the legal system. There, as nowhere else, the question turns on society's legal obligations. In general, it appears as if there is less controversy about discontinuation of dialysis than that of stopping medical feeding and hydration in the irreversibly incompetent patient. In the eyes of the courts and public, the 'high-tec' aspects of dialysis appear to put it in a separate class from parenteral feeding. Finally, two of us attempt an ethical analysis of the morality of stopping treatment, examined from the different viewpoints of Kantian deontology, consequentialism, recognition of virtue, human mutual interdependency and existentialism.

For the final section, we invited physicians and philosophers from India, Africa, Japan, Eastern Europe, Great Britain and China to contribute self-chosen topics from their experiences in these different parts of the world. In an interesting clash of opinion, Reddy and Mani, both writing from India, reach diametrically opposite conclusions on the moral consequences of commerce in kidneys, a practice that is perhaps more common there than elsewhere. From Africa, Barsoum writes about the dilemmas a Western-trained nephrologist faces when confronted by the technological imperative of dialysis in economic conflict with other un-met public health needs. He believes that, in Egypt more than elsewhere, power governs the selection of patients for treatment. We respectfully disagree with his view. The problem of inequality based on power is timeless and universal. The first written words of mankind from Lagesh by King Urakigina, 5000 years ago promises 'my laws are against exploitation of the poor'. We have a long way to go.

Atsumi tries to explain the immense paradox of the Japanese acceptance of dialysis but spurning of transplantation. Somehow, the mixture of Buddhism, Shintoism, paternalism and distrust of the medical profession has led to the rejection of organ donation by the population at large. Valek then gives the view from Eastern Europe where money is scarce, and medical technology not favoured by the state. He describes the problems posed by faulty equipment and outmoded technology, resulting in the spread of communicable diseases such as hepatitis, in conjunction with a selection process which physicians allowed to be largely governed by the sole parameter of outcome. The order of the day seems to be: Select the young, especially only those with primary renal disease, and try to throttle back on dialysis so that transplantation can keep up with the acceptance rate to dialysis.

The situation in Great Britain, perhaps the only country which has openly acknowledged the reality of economic constraints, is given by Anthony Wing. When patients were few, physicians were 'unfettered by financial constraint' and politicians greedily credited themselves for a healthcare service which they happily termed the 'jewel in the crown of the welfare state'. When money was not forthcoming, acceptance rates in Great Britain seriously lagged behind acceptance rates elsewhere in the West. The situation was bitterly denounced in the press by patients and physicians, but no general public outcry occurred. One wonders about the virtue of solidarity when Wing writes that 'the people had been accustomed to rationing, having lived on an island under siege. The professions had inherited a status in society which allowed them to adopt a paternalistic attitude to making life and death decisions for an unquestioning public, and even the politicians believed their own rhetoric' [!]. Now, with a change of political fortune, the market approach is said to have arrived for the National Health Service. We will have to wait and see what will transpire there, as the system follows the American paradigm but the money is no longer abundant. Wing describes how physicians in Great Britain, with a mixture of despair, ingenuity and perhaps moral blinders, try to cope with scarcity in supplying their patients with those necessities which the countries around them seem to be able to supply to their patients.

Finally, Ren-Zong Qiu from the Institute of Philosophy at the Chinese Academy of Social Sciences, gives the Chinese perspective on these expensive high-tec procedures. Oddly, perhaps, he concludes that individuals have to take a back seat for the overall societal good. 'A man of humanity will never seek to live at the expense of injuring humanity. He would rather sacrifice his life in order to realize humanity'. He also falls back on Confucianism and Taoism in claiming that 'life and death are the chance of Heaven; wealth and honour depend on Heaven', coupled with a principle of non-action ('Wu Wei'). The latter does not mean 'do nothing', but rather do nothing unnatural or beyond nature. Professor Qiu uses this as an explanation why 'some Chinese who insist on traditional values reject dialysis and transplantation, even when a clinical situation is critical and the quality of life would be improved by treatment.'

So, there they are, these sometimes perplexing and contradictory views, principles, rules, solutions and suggestions from those we asked either to look at problems from above or to give experiences derived from the struggle itself, below. Neither of us is naive enough to believe that blueprints exist, but here at least many issues are out on the table together with the complexities of trying to solve them. Essentially, there are only three reactions one can take while looking at them: deny their existence, enforce one's own solution by a moral warfare, or try to understand each other. Perhaps even moral strangers can come to a reasonable agreement of what our actions should be.

PART ONE

The principles

1. The search for a universal system of ethics: post-modern disappointments and contemporary possibilities

H. TRISTRAM ENGELHARDT, JR.

I. Can ethics provide moral authority for health care policy?

One raises philosophical questions regarding issues of ethics and justice in the hope of disclosing guiding criteria for judgment and action. Because of the diversity of human interests, inclinations, and moral visions, such questioning leads to disputes about proper policy and conduct. Such disputes are often characterized by conflicting judgments about what behavior is morally opprobrious and what should be forcefully interdicted. This is nowhere more true than with regard to the use of the human body. Religions and traditional cultures have appropriately regarded the human body as a unique object of moral and aesthetic concern. It is our place in the world. Because the body is special, many religions and cultures have rules against its commercial use.[1] These traditional concerns, often expressed in prohibitions against prostitution, cast their light and shadow across discussions regarding the sale of human organs. Terms such as 'exploitation' and 'commercialization', for example, are introduced to build a case against selling organs. Such concerns, along with life-and-death decisions faced in initiating, withdrawing, and paying for dialysis, make this an area of choice laden with moral interests and controversies.

One would hope to show what rational men and women ought to establish as policy in the area of dialysis and the acquisition of organs. Were one able to achieve this goal, one could establish what constitutes both rational policy and moral policy and dismiss those in disagreement as being irrational. In particular, if it could be shown what rational persons as such *should* endorse regarding dialysis and the sale of organs, the use of coercive force in the realization of public policy would find coincident moral and rational foundations. If this project could be successfully completed, the use of coercion to enforce rationally justified health care policies would not be alien to the true nature of those on whom it was visited, for it would be achieving what rational individuals should endorse. It is inviting to hope that one can in general secular rational terms justify a content-full universal system of ethics. The difficulty, however, is that this project appears impossible to complete.

Two indications of the difficulty should be noted from the start. First, there is considerable content-full disagreement regarding matters of ethics, if one examines

3

C. M. Kjellstrand and J. B. Dossetor (eds): Ethical Problems in Dialysis and Transplantation, 3–19.
© 1992 *Kluwer Academic Publishers. Printed in the Netherlands.*

the fine grain of disputes. Though there are moral fashions and passions of political correctness so that at times few will openly admit their moral doubts in certain areas, still, when one plumbs matters in detail and with persistence, considerable substantive disagreement is found. It may be claimed, for example, that there is general agreement that one should not murder. Yet, when one considers what should count as murder, disagreement emerges. One need only consider as an illustration the question as to whether abortion should count as an instance of murder. The debate regarding the moral propriety of selling organs provides another example.

Secondly, disputes in ethics generally go on and on without conclusive resolution. Such disputes do not turn centrally on disputes regarding matters of logic. Thus, agreement concerning a common logical system or framework will not be sufficient to resolve moral disputes. Nor are matters of moral dispute merely matters of debate regarding facts, unless one recognizes that the facts have already been clothed with moral significance. In actual everyday discussions, facts have already taken on a moral coloration or valuation, such that, if one is having a moral dispute within a particular moral community, the facts often not only speak for themselves, but, since they are value-laden, they can frequently resolve moral controversies [5]. When individuals meet from different moral or metaphysical perspectives, that is, with different views about how to value the facts or about the deep significance of the facts, the disputes tend to be interminable. In an important sense, the disputants in such circumstances do not see the facts in the same way. Indeed, they do not share the same facts, for matters appear clothed with different moral and metaphysical judgments and expectations. This circumstance is again illustrated by the controversies regarding the moral significance of abortion. Individuals who share metaphysical and moral principles can agree with each other but persist in disagreeing with those who fall beyond the communality of mutual assumptions. In particular, there are no decisive 'facts' regarding the beginning of life to which individuals who lack common moral and metaphysical assumptions can appeal to resolve their debates regarding the morality of abortion. As we will see, the same is the case regarding many of the issues such as the sale of organs and the availability of dialysis.

This difficulty in achieving a rationally grounded resolution of moral debates constitutes a profound embarrassment not only for ethics but for public policy and health care policy, and appears as a moral crisis against the background of prior expectations. The European Middle Ages bequeathed a robust model of morally justified coercive public authority: appeals were made to divine authority and its authorization of the civic institutions of the time. Those institutions that acted with divine authority and in concord with the established beliefs of the Christian West were seen to function not simply coercively, but to use coercion with moral justification. Justification in terms of faith was intertwined with a faith in reason and the ability of reason to secure a rational grounding for much that was endorsed within the framework of the regnant religion. Central to the European modernity that developed after the collapse of the Christian synthesis of the Middle Ages was the attempt to justify a secular ethics and public policy, which in many ways resembled the ethics and public policy of the Middle Ages, only devoid of a direct appeal to the Christian God, and cleansed of some of the particularities of Christian commitment. The hope was to have much of Christian conviction with regard to public authority and morality without a reliance on the Christian God. Philosophical postmodernity can be described as the realization that this project cannot be successful [7]. This realization has profound implications for the development of morally authoritative health care policy bearing on dialysis and transplantation: there is no content-full universal secular ethics.

This embarrassment of moral theory is not unanticipated. The difficulties have been fairly clear since the end of the 19th and the beginning of the 20th century. Indeed, reflections on these difficulties have led to disquietude and reassessments of the status of ethics by philosophers engaged in theoretical ethics.[2] What is interesting is that little notice has been taken within applied ethics of these concerns about the status of moral claims [6]. Still, the failure to face this difficulty is only too understandable: these concerns bring into question much of contemporary bioethics and the ethics of health care planning. The challenge is to face these unpleasant difficulties and to secure some secular moral foundation for contemporary bioethics and the ethics of health care planning. If this challenge is to be met, it will be necessary on the one hand to take seriously the diversity of human moral visions, while on the other hand finding a common moral fabric. There is real disagreement among men and women of developed moral reflection regarding the morality of selling organs. That diversity must be acknowledged. At the same time, one must find a foundational moral communality in terms of which secular health care policy can be justified.

II. The impossibility of discovering content for a universal secular ethics

The moral challenge is to choose authoritatively among alternative policy options. Since evaluations of states of affairs depend significantly on the rankings or weightings given to different outcomes or circumstances, one must know how to rank or weight outcomes or circumstances. To accomplish this, one must already know how to evaluate outcomes or circumstances. The circle is vicious. It is not possible to identify an account of moral rationality, a way of assessing consequences, or a content-full hypothetical choice theory without already begging the question that is at stake. For example, to assess the consequences of different approaches to the donation or sale of organs, one must be able to determine the sum of liberty consequences, equality consequences, and health consequences of different policy options, but to make such an assessment, one must know how to rank considerations of liberty, equality, and health. Nor will it do simply to endorse that approach which will lead to the greatest preference satisfaction. One will first need to have decided not only how to weight present and future preferences but also rational versus impassioned preferences, in order to identify the approach which maximizes preference satisfaction. This choice, though, cannot be made on the basis of consequences without begging the question.

Similarly, an appeal to a disinterested observer will be equally useless. If the observer is truly disinterested, it will not provide a basis for a choice among various approaches to the donation or sale of organs. If a choice is provided, it is because one has fitted out the hypothetical decision-maker or hypothetical contractors with a particular thin theory of the good, moral sense, or understanding of moral rationality. However, it is just this that was at stake to begin with. Nor are there normative facts of human nature outside of particular moral understandings. Regarded outside of any particular moral viewpoint, human nature is the outcome of random mutations, selective pressures, genetic drift, various catastrophic events, and the constraints set by chemical and physical structures. Any understanding of successful human adaptation depends on the goals chosen or recognized by individuals, but the choice among goals is exactly what is at question. In short, there is no way to turn into reason itself or to 'examine the facts' in order to discover the correct content-full account of ethics.

Many ethical disputes are resistant to resolution, and a major crisis looms, as has been noted, regarding the justification of content-full health care policy. When individuals committed to different rankings of important human goals or values dispute regarding the propriety or impropriety of different policies, as, for example, with respect to the donation or sale of organs, they will not be able in general secular terms to discover the correct policy. There will be quite different views of what is at stake. Those who rank liberty interests highly may regard those who would forbid the sale of organs as exploiting individuals in the service of one among many alternative understandings of human excellence by forbidding individuals from selling their organs, so that those who oppose commercialization can feel morally satisfied. On the other hand, those who have moral intuitions adverse to commercializing the transfer of organs will see such liberty interests outweighed by the importance of preventing the commercial provision of organs, and will regard those who agree to sell their organs as being exploited by those purchasing.

This contrast of moral viewpoints can be stark. Those who value liberty highly may regard those opposed to the sale of organs as deeply perverse. They may consider such individuals as thwarting the opportunities of individuals to free themselves from impoverishment in order to satisfy a wide range of preferences through the sale of their organs. Supporters of organ sales may agree that certain protections must be set in place to avoid fraudulent agreements, but they will not recognize the legitimacy of the special moral intuitions of those who hold that the commercialization of organs is *per se* evil. On the other hand, those who regard sentiments against commercialization as straightforwardly conclusive will consider those who favor the sale of organs as lacking in proper moral sensibilities. Because of their fundamentally different ways of ranking consequences and assessing moral choices, partisans of these two different approaches will be unable to find grounds for common agreement. The dispute will be potentially interminable, somewhat in the nature of fundamental religious disagreements.

Worse yet, if there is no basis for rationally choosing one view over the other, then in general secular terms any one particular policy option is, in principle, no more rational than its rivals. This will mean that the choice of a particular policy of either proscribing or allowing the sale of organs cannot be justified as the one to be endorsed by reasonable men and women. The choice, instead, takes on a particularistic character: the choice reflects the prior endorsement of one particular, but from a general secular arbitrary viewpoint, understanding of proper human behavior. This example confronts us with the parochial character of the moral content in secular ethics.

One cannot establish particular canonical moral content outside of a specific religious, ideological, or moral tradition. Outside of certain moral communities and their particular accounts or narratives about human flourishing and well-being, there is no canonical, content-full account of appropriate moral conduct. This circumstance is what Lyotard has characterized as the post-modern predicament. 'The grand narrative has lost its credibility, regardless of what mode of unification it uses, regardless of whether it is a speculative narrative or a narrative of emancipation.' The choice of a particular moral narrative involves an act of conversion, submission, or identification. One assumes a particular history and/or a particular account of the human condition. What one does not find is a universal content-full morality or a universal content-full account of human well-being and flourishing. This failure to secure canonical content for secular ethics is the source of great difficulty for international statements regarding the moral probity or immorality of different approaches to the donation or sale of organs. Such statements lack a justification in a universal content-full ethics.

III. The language of moral strangers: a content-less universal secular ethic

In a world where there are individuals with consciences informed by different moral viewpoints or narratives, there is still the possibility of peaceable cooperation by an appeal to a moral standpoint that each can understand as binding, even on moral strangers. The term 'moral strangers' is introduced to identify individuals who in particular moral controversies do not share sufficient common assumptions to enable them to conclude their debate on the basis of sound rational arguments. The term 'moral strangers' contrasts with 'moral friends' who share sufficient moral premises to allow a controversy at hand to be resolved by rational argument. The same individuals may, depending on the moral controversy with which they are engaged, be either moral friends or moral strangers. The former may have the special advantage of being able to resolve controversies because they share content-full moral assumptions that allows them to appeal to an accepted moral authority.

The distinction between moral friends and moral strangers underscores why it is misguided to expect the kinds of resolutions to debates that occur among moral friends to be available for the controversies shared by moral strangers. In particular, controversies about the moral probity of human organ sales or about what should count as justice in the distribution of health care resources, are difficult for moral strangers to resolve, precisely because they do not share common moral intuitions about the importance of liberty or the offensiveness of selling organs. Still, even when they do not share common moral assumptions, a kind of common moral fabric of collaboration can be both presupposed and established. Insofar as one is interested in resolving controversies other than through a direct appeal to force, and even when individuals do not share a common moral understanding by the grace of God, history, or ideological commitment, and despite the moral vacuity or indeterminacy of general secular moral rationality, one can still frame a common fabric of moral action on the basis of mutual agreement. The commitment to resolving issues peaceably, albeit as moral strangers, will mean that individuals can act together with common agreement, drawing authority from that agreement, realizing that, when there is collaboration with moral strangers, moral authority cannot be derived from appeals to God, history, or reason.

In this circumstance, no moral content is necessary to assure the existence of a common fabric of moral authority. It is enough to recognize that anyone who uses another without consent sets aside the one basis for common, peaceable, morally authoritative action when moral strangers meet. Such a secular moral outlaw falls beyond the secular moral pale in being deprived of a secular justification for protesting against punitive and defensive force. On the other hand, those who collaborate can recognize that their common endeavors have moral authority in the simple and straightforward sense that they have received common authorization. As a consequence, in the moral context of post-modernity, the salient moral institutions are properly limited democracies, the free market, and free and informed consent, because they draw their authority from those who participate in these practices, and do not require any foundational metaphysical, religious, or moral assumptions.

To visualize better the limited moral authority of limited democracies, the readers of this essay might imagine what it would be to bring them together in order to form a government, and then determine the morality of organ sales or the character of justice in health care distribution. It is likely that the readers will include individuals of diverse religious, cultural, and political persuasions. Insofar as this is the case, they will not share a common understanding of the good life or the moral purposes of governmental structures. Despite this lack of agreement, they can agree to act together with mutual authorization, as long as those who participate are not used without their permission, and insofar as common endeavors conform to the agreements of those who decide to participate. This point of departure makes individuals central, not because individuals are valued, but because individuals are the starting point of democratic authorization when one cannot appeal to common understandings of God, the significance of history, or the content of morality. It is enough to understand that one may not touch, use, or employ others without their permission and that, given common agreement, limited but complex social undertakings are possible.

The point is that the fabric of secular morality and the moral basis for secular health care policy do not collapse if one honestly faces the post-modern moral predicament. One does not need a transcendent ground or a canonical content-full account of ethics to authorize the use of defensive or punitive force against those who commit murder, battery, burglary, or rape. The enforcement of recorded contracts can be given authority by democratic agreement. Most importantly, there will be the possibility to create welfare entitlements of various sorts, including the provision of dialysis. One does not need to agree on a concrete universal narrative in order to provide police protection against most criminal activities, or to establish by democratic choice a web of refusable welfare rights. One can develop a rather robust account of governmental authority without solving the post-modern predicament, without denying the obvious, namely, that there is no content-full universal moral narrative that can serve as the basis for, or the expression of, a universal content-full ethics. A secular government can be formed and given authority to use common resources in accord with established democratic procedures, even if no particular religious or other content-full understanding of distributive justice may be established (i.e., consent for such cannot be presumed), and the ways in which individuals choose to use their own organs by themselves or with consenting others, falls beyond the authority of the state. Without explicit agreement, one cannot assume that the readers would have conveyed authority over their bodies to the government.[3]

One can in fact concede much to the emotivists and logical positivists and still rescue a universal ethics as a construct of peaceable wills. One will not be able to give a transcendent justification for having a peaceable will, nor will there be general moral considerations to motivate such an act of will. But those who do engage in this enterprise of peaceably fashioning secular moral authority will be able to recognize a universal moral fabric without presupposing any particular content-full moral premises, while at the same time rationally disarming any who reject this fabric of any general secular grounds for protesting against defensive or punitive force. Somewhat like empirical science, which does not require a metaphysical agreement, only the interest in empirically resolving intersubjectively certain disputes concerning phenomenal reality, this approach to morality provides a practice open and available for moral strangers without presupposing any metaphysical assumptions or content-full moral premises.

The result is that one salvages much of modern philosophy's moral project, and in doing so, provides the basis for a universal secular moral framework, even if one cannot disclose a content-full universal ethic. One justifies something like a *jus naturale*, a basic moral fabric that binds all who ask the secular moral question of how moral strangers can peaceably collaborate. Moral restrictions can be justified (e.g., one may not take organs from individuals without their authorization) and moral entitlements can be created (one can agree to provide dialysis out of communal funds for those in need). The difficulty is that one does not find the moral authority to forbid consensual acts among agreeing adults, such as the agreement to sell an organ.

IV. The peaceable creation of a universal secular moral framework

Though at first blush these philosophical explorations might suggest a world quite different from the one in which most of us live, many of these reflections in fact show how to reconstruct the moral structures that support the successful moral practices of the contemporary world, including the central goals of contemporary health care policy. People have substantial moral disagreements regarding matters of moral substance. Yet, they peaceably collaborate in large-scale undertakings, despite these differences. Those institutions that function with the clearest moral warrants under such circumstances of moral diversity and disagreement are those that presuppose no content-full understanding of human flourishing, but instead allow peaceable individuals with diverse moral visions to collaborate as far as they are able and interested, and to maintain their integrity when their conscience forbids joining in particular endeavors. It is for this reason, as has already been noted, that limited democracies and the free market constitute the triumphant political forms at the end of the 20th century. These institutions have succeeded, not so much because individuals share a common vision of the good life, liberty, fairness, justice, or exploitation, but because they require no such presuppositions. In particular, limited democracies require minimal substantive moral agreement, while allowing large-scale collaboration. A limited democracy enables much to be done communally, while recognizing a robust place for private choices and undertakings, because it recognizes the difference between public and private morality. Indeed, in a limited democracy, individuals can live their lives within content-full private moral communities of religious and political commitment, which might be totalitarian if they were allowed to determine the regnant morality of the state.

Given the limitations of secular moral reasoning and of secular moral authority, health care policy must be framed in ways that draw authority from the consent of those involved. It can generally presuppose limited albeit diverse commitments to human solidarity and to protecting others from harm. These circumstances will allow developing health care policy in general, and policy concerning the use of dialysis and organ transplantation in particular, around three major moral principles.

A. *The principle of authorization*

Insofar as is feasible, those engaged in collaborative enterprises should be able to show that they have the agreement of their collaborators. Limited democracies should be able to demonstrate the consent of their citizens. Markets should be able to show the consent of those who engage in transactions.[4] In health care policy, the accent should be on the development of practices that support the free consent of patients, and which do not interfere in the peaceable, consensual activity of competent individuals. The principle of authorization will in many ways appear similar to what others have referred to as a principle of autonomy. However, the principle of authorization does not endorse a special value for liberty or for autonomous action. It quite readily accepts the circumstance that many individuals in many cultures and contexts may prefer physicians and other health care workers who, in a fiduciary paternalism,[5] achieve their good without frightening disclosures of grim prognoses or onerous recountings of distant and unlikely risks.

The difference between the principle of autonomy and the principle of authorization is significant in a world populated by different cultures and different concrete moral expectations, where one cannot presume that all patients wish to live as isolated individuals and be treated outside the moral confines of their families and concrete social commitments. In many cultures, patients are quite pleased that family members and/or physicians will negotiate many of the choices regarding their treatment. The principle of authorization does not suggest that one ought to constrain individuals within traditional societies to revalue their social arrangements and face medical and moral decisions in the same ways that most individuals do in the United States. The principle of authorization does not require valuing liberty first, but rather that one respect the choice to exit from enveloping social structures and be self-determining. The principle of authorization protects freedom without giving a special value to individualistic autonomy. A consequence of the difference between the principle of authorization with its focus on respecting individual choice, and the principle of autonomy with the value it gives to individualistic choice, is that complicated consent forms, as one finds in the United States, need not, as a matter of moral obligation, be exported to all in the world. Such consent forms should in principle be available for those who would wish them. In many societies, though, it should be more than sufficient to ensure that people know of their availability.

B. *The principle of limited protection*

Out of concerns such as self-protection, solidarity, and altruism, most societies will decide to protect individuals who might be harmed by fraud or coercion. Such protective practices and institutions, which can be established out of a variety of moral and other interests, are particularly important for endeavors such as the acquisition of organs, especially when financial and other inducements are offered. However, such protection must be limited by the principle of authorization: individuals who competently decline protection should not receive it. This limitation does not spring from any particular value given to freedom, but from the circumstance that secular authority is derived from individual consent, such that a claim that one may protect the best interests of others will be defeated if individuals refuse protection. On the other hand, protective institutions do not need to presume any particular content-full view of proper moral conduct in order to find justification. It is enough to note that it is likely that human interests will usually be sufficient for the political creation of protective institutions that will draw their moral authority from the limited democracies that fashion them.

C. *The principle of limited solidarity*

From various concerns, such as self-protection, solidarity, and altruism, most societies will create limited social insurance policies against losses at the natural and social lotteries. Again, one need not seek justification in a background common sense of beneficence or justice. Rather, the political orchestration of various moral and non-moral sentiments will generally lead to the social creation of civil entitlements to health care. In affluent countries, this is likely to include limited entitlements to dialysis and organ transplantation. But such entitlements must be understood as created, limited entitlements, since there are as many theories of justice, beneficence, and altruism as there are major religions. Instead of deriving a content-full view of the just provision of dialysis or organ transplantation from some background philosophical theory of justice, fairness, or beneficence, entitlements to health care should in general secular terms be regarded as political creations that derive their moral authority from the activities of limited democracies. Given the failure to discover *the* canonical account of fairness, justice, or beneficence, and given the limited moral authority of limited democracies, the public creation of entitlements should not prejudice the possibility of private entitlements coming into existence, either through private insurance or private market transactions. Limited democracies are constrained to live with both public and private tiers of health care in that they will not in principle be able to show that all resources are publicly owned, nor can they show that individuals may not purchase additional care with their private resources after having paid their taxes ([4], pp. 336–374). To hold that all resources are communal or that citizens may be constrained to live according to a particular content-full notion of egalitarianism or justice, would require discovering a canonical content-full understanding of moral rationality, which is not possible.

V. The rules of bioethics: moral conduct of health care in a secular, morally pluralist context

The secular moral principles of authorization, limited protection, and limited solidarity are forwarded as guides for health care policy, given the limits of secular moral reasoning. Far from wishing to undermine moral visions and concerns, this approach is offered in order to provide the strongest case for the most robust web of moral obligations that can be justified universally, that is, outside of particular religious, political, or ideological contexts. Those who live their moral lives within the content-full moral contexts of particular religious or ideological commitments will feel a loss of substance and an absence of direction. This is unavoidable if one attempts to deal morally, not with moral friends, but with moral strangers.

In this post-modern context, deprived of the content of traditional moral frameworks, and against a plurality of visions of justice, fairness, and rights in health care, basic moral rules of thumb can still be articulated to guide physicians, other health care professionals, and health care policy-makers. These rules of thumb can somewhat procrusteanly and tendentiously be stated in a decalogue.

A. *Gain specific authorization through consent*

Since the authorization to use individuals as patients comes from those individuals, one should acquire from them as clear and specific a permission as possible in order to guide treatment. The problems that arise as a result of ambiguities regarding the wishes of patients can often be cured simply by asking patients what they want. Since patients provide authorization for treatment, they can remove authorization for treatment.

B. *Plan ahead: use advance directives*

Because all patients will die, and because many will be incompetent prior to death, it is important to inquire of patients how they wish to be treated when incompetent, who should make judgments on their behalf, and the circumstances under which treatment should be withdrawn. It will often be helpful in discussing such matters to distinguish the difference between appointing a proxy decision-maker for periods of incompetence from the subject of deciding what treatment to withhold or withdraw in the face of terminal illness. Frequently, both physicians and patients will find it more acceptable to discuss who should make decisions in the event of periods of incompetency, even if this discussion encompasses making decisions in the face of death, than straightforwardly to address planning for terminal illness. It will be helpful to learn as much as possible regarding the wishes of patients, in order to give direction to both proxy decision-makers and physicians faced with the decision of limiting treatment in the face of either death or severe deterioration of quality of life [3]. Finally, in most countries and cultures it will be important to establish either by law or custom, presumptive proxy decision-makers (e.g., spouses and other family members) who may make decisions about limiting and directing care, should the patient become incompetent. Such practices put individuals on notice that, should they wish to have other than customary proxy decision-makers, they should take steps to appoint them. Advance directives are of importance for the decision to provide dialysis, for often one must contemplate initiating treatment when the patient is incompetent, quality of life circumscribed, and/or the possibility of death considerable. The agreement to provide organs for donation at death can be regarded as a special instance of an advance directive, one reaching out to cover one's body after death.

C. *Withdrawing treatment is, ceteris paribus, the same as withholding treatment*

In general secular moral terms, no essential difference can be discovered between withdrawing a treatment and withholding a treatment. In either case, the usual justifications will be the lack of the patient's permission (or that of the patient's surrogate or proxy), or a decision to limit access to a particular resource. In the first case, the lack of authority to treat the patient is as decisive in the case of withdrawing treatment as in the case of withholding. In the second case, the matter turns on the circumstance that entitlements to goods and services are always limited created entitlements. In health care, entitlements to goods and services tend properly to be fashioned, taking into account the costs involved, the likely ratio of benefits over harms, and the alternative projects in which one could engage. However, if there are special cultural or other concerns that cause withdrawal to appear to be morally different from withholding treatment, these experiences of differences, because they constitute socially and psychologically engendered benefits and harms, need to be considered in framing policy. Finally, there may be significant costs to patients if it is not as easy to withdraw a treatment as to withhold it. In this instance a bias may develop against providing treatment, in the fear that once it is begun, it cannot be terminated. Such a circumstance would have the adverse consequence of discouraging physicians and institutions from providing a trial of treatment.

D. *The right to refuse care; different from the right to demand care*

Individuals require only themselves in order to refuse treatment with moral authority. Individuals require agreements, commitments, or common moral understandings shared with others in order to demand treatment with moral right. The right to refuse treatment is in contrast a forbearance right, justified in the core of the secular morality that binds moral strangers. If one touches or otherwise uses individuals without their permission, one sets aside the very possibility of peaceably resolving moral controversies in the absence of unambiguously understood revelations from God, and in the absence of canonical, content-full, secular, moral rationality. To make claims against others for their goods and services requires a common understanding of why those others are morally obliged to be forthcoming. Such moral obligations can in secular terms be created only by agreement or common understanding. As a consequence, there is a deep asymmetry between the right to refuse medical treatments such as hemodialysis and organ transplantation, and the right to demand such treatment. For the right to demand such treatments to have secular moral standing, it must be made within a system of created entitlements that includes the treatments at stake.

E. *Entitlements are created, not discovered, and therefore should be clarified by stipulation*

Misunderstandings regarding the scope of entitlements to treatments such as hemodialysis and organ transplantation can be reduced by specifying as clearly as possible the circumstances under which the services will be available. In the absence of a canonical secular moral vision, one will not be able to discover how to translate particular needs or interests into rights to health care. Such a translation can only occur through the societal or contractual creation of limited entitlements to health care goods and services. Since entitlements to health care services are created, they can therefore be fashioned with clarity. In the structuring of such entitlements, depending on prior social agreements, groups including limited democracies may properly take into account such considerations as costs, likelihood of success, and even age. In addition, when creating entitlements, groups should, out of prudence, include provision for the authoritative resolution of disputes and ambiguities (e.g., by use of hospital ethics committees). Such clarifications constitute the analogue to advance directives with respect to entitlements to treatments. Here, however, it is usually the social entity that creates the entitlements which must then in advance specify the scope and character of the entitlements created.

F. *Favor the language of solidarity over the language of justice*

Because there are as many theories of justice, fairness, and rights to health care as there are major religions, and because the languages of justice, fairness, and rights to health care tend to convey a tone of moral righteousness that cannot be grounded in general secular moral terms, one should seek moral frameworks in which to articulate entitlements to health care services, such as hemodialysis and organ transplantation, which do not support absolutist claims that can lead to unwarranted coercive intervention. Instead, the moral discourse that develops around considerations of limited solidarity or social insurance can come closer for general secular ethics to accounting for political structures with general secular warrant: in creating health care entitlements, societies are endorsing one among many other possible responses to losses at the natural and social lotteries. Because social entitlements to health care are properly created out of common resources, and because the secular moral authority of governments is limited, individuals will retain a fundamental right by default to use their private goods and services to purchase additional health care (including hemodialysis and organ transplantation), by direct payments or through private health care insurance. Particular egalitarian views or ideologies may not, with secular moral authority, justify forbidding a private tier of access to such health care. Again, this is the case not because such private health care is helpful, useful, or to be valued, but rather because of the limits of secular moral reasoning and secular moral authority.

16

On the one hand, for various reasons individuals may join together in governmental projects of assisting the impecunious in ways that will appear to constitute a policy of an egalitarianism of altruism. That is, it will appear to be an attempt to make all equal by advantaging those with limited resources, but it will most fundamentally be a policy authorized by a limited democracy about how to use communal resources. Some citizens will regard such activities as altruistic undertakings, others as attempts to build political coalitions, etc. On the other hand, a government may not coercively pursue a policy of an egalitarianism of envy, which forbids citizens to use the resources available to them after paying their taxes to purchase additional goods and services beyond the basic package created through social convention. The limits of governmental moral authority and the existence of private property will constitute moral barriers against such totalitarian claims regarding private goods and services (i.e., that they may be totally claimed for majoritarian moral projects). Two tiers of health care entitlements will come naturally into existence as a function of human finitude: the finitude of human resources, the outcomes of the natural and social lotteries, and the limited moral authority of secular social and political institutions.

G. *Protect rights to privacy*

Rights to privacy exist by default. Rights to privacy as moral rights are a function of the limited moral authority of social agreements, in particular, the limited moral authority of governments. Because limited democracies receive from their citizens at best limited authority over the peaceable undertakings of those citizens with consenting others, wide ranges of exclaves from governmental and societal interference will exist not because these are valued, but because one cannot justify governmental intrusion. In order coercively to intervene with moral authority and without consent, one must be able to show that what is done is correct and that one has the moral right to act over the protests of those visited with the coercion. These conditions will in principle not be able to be met where a common canonical understanding of proper actions and deportment cannot be discovered. The right to refuse treatment, the right to have treatment withdrawn, the right to use one's body as one wishes with consenting others, and the right to use one's private property as one wishes with consenting others, are rights justified not in some positive picture of human flourishing, but in terms of the limits of secular moral authority.

H. *Commercialization of organ transfers not per se wrong*

In the absence of an appeal to a particular religious or ideological understanding of the proper role of commerce in organs and bodies, there will not be a way to determine when commercial trade in human organs is morally improper. The attempt coercively to forbid individuals from selling their organs will appear in secular terms as a form of exploitation by individuals who feel morally distressed if others sell their organs. Therefore, in order to protect themselves from this distress, such individuals will be tempted to use state force to forbid those who wish to advantage themselves by selling their organs. But this moral claim or the authority coercively to realize it cannot be secured in general secular terms.

I. *Establish protections against abuse*

The history of mankind is replete with venality, overreaching, and the use of fraud and coercion giving substantial motivation for establishing protective practices and institutions. Nowhere has this been more true in recent history than in terms of the governmental coercive oppression of citizens. One might think here in particular of the abuses undertaken by Nazi experimentation. One would need as well to recognize as an example the systematic difficulties in the health care system of the Soviet Union and its dramatic adverse impact on its citizens [8]. The impropriety of fraud and coercion in health care can be understood outside of appeals to a particular content-full view of morality, because the fraudulent or forcible use of individuals is a rejection of the practice of interaction among moral strangers in commonly justifiable ways and without fundamental reliance on force. Physicians and other health care workers may quite properly take steps to develop policies to insure that neither governments, corporations, health care institutions, nor individual practitioners abuse patients by fraud or coercive practices or interventions.

J. *Acknowledge the radical difference between general secular morality and the morality of particular religious and ideological commitments*

Many individuals live in robust moral communities framed by strong religious and ideological commitments. In terms of their concrete moral commitments, such individuals will often have grounds for holding what others do to be wrong, though they will not be able to demonstrate the wrongness in general secular terms. They will feel a tension between the secular language that peaceably binds moral strangers and their own content-full moral commitments. They will often find themselves in the position of holding that an individual has a secular right to engage in activities they know to be wrong in special religious or ideological terms. As a consequence, they will find themselves holding that 'individuals have the right (in the sense that general secular arguments cannot justify the use of interdicting force) to sell their organs for transplantation, but it is wrong (e.g., "I know it to be wrong in terms of my religious and/or ideological commitments").' Still others may refuse to join in the project of resolving disputes peaceably in terms that can be justified to moral strangers in general secular terms. For them, nothing can be said that will be convincing, though in general secular terms they are the proper recipients of punitive and defensive force.[6]

VI. Universal morality in the post-modern world

The 20th century has seen the political failure of numerous ideologies bent on discovering content-full understandings of human history and human flourishing. It has witnessed the increasing secularization and diminishing salience of Western Christianity in Europe[7] and the large scale of abandonment of Marxist metaphysics in the former Soviet bloc countries. Systems that claim by reason to disclose content-full general moral foundations have collapsed as major social undertakings. This history confronts the bioethicist with the particularist character of much moral content. An examination of the capacities of moral reasoning reveal that one cannot discover in general secular terms *the* canonical content-full understanding of morality. Moral content cannot be found in reason or through examining the character of the world. One must always bring to the interpretation of the world moral expectations before one can see moral facts.[8] There is no secular content-full universal morality. Yet this does not leave morality politics or health care policy in the hands of nihilism or an unqualified relativism. There is still a foundation for building a universal fabric of mutual respect binding moral strangers in a post-modern world. This foundation sustains the moral authority of limited democracies, free and informed consent, and the free market. It springs from individuals and creates communities. In the absence of a secular, content-full, canonical morality and against a plurality of moral visions, individuals can authorize common moral projects and give them an ethical standing that can bind moral strangers. There remains a contentless, yet universal ethic to guide health care policy.

Notes

1. It must be observed that a number of religions and cultures included temple prostitution, so that the sale of intimate relations, as an anthropological phenomenon, has not generally been seen to be improper.
2. The problem of establishing the truth value, if any, for secular moral claims has been discussed widely. See, for example, [1] and [14]. The problems that beset moral philosophy have dramatic implications for the possibility of making sense of what it would mean to have a rationally justified resolution of public policy controversies. For an overview of some of the questions and difficulties involved in the project of bringing justified closure to public policy debates possessing a value overlay, see [5]. Recent discussions of 'post-modernity' or 'after philosophy' indicate a significant difficulty for the project of selecting in other than an arbitrary fashion among many public policy choices. For some recent reflections in philosophical post-modernity, see, for example, [2], [7], [10], [12], and [13]. Alasdair MacIntyre's *Whose Justice? Which Rationality?* suggests the difficulty of selecting among rival understandings of justice and of moral rationality. See [11].
3. Because secular moral authority cannot be justified in terms of a particular religious or content-full philosophical view, authority is derived from the consent of persons. Therefore, the authority of persons over themselves is always primary and central, while the property status of mere things must in some fashion be derived from the actions and consent of individuals. The result is that rights to privacy are primordial and limit the authority of the state, while claims to real property involve others and therefore conventions established by states. See, for example, [4], pp. 104–156.

4. Given the centrality of the principle of peaceable authorization, consent in the circumstances of market transaction will be valid in the absence of fraud or coercion on the part of the participants in the particular transaction. That nature or third parties have disadvantaged participants in a market transaction will not invalidate the transaction because no particular ranking of liberty or autonomy can be made to remove the moral justification conveyed by authorization.

5. A distinction must be drawn between strong paternalism in which some individuals claim to have the right, because of the overriding good at stake, to act to achieve the best interests of others, contrary to their wishes, versus forms of paternalism that derive their authority from the consent of those treated. In medicine, what is often at stake is a form of implicit fiduciary paternalism. That is, the social circumstances clearly give evidence of the patient's implicit permission having been conveyed by the patient to a physician to act on behalf of the patient's good.

6. This essay sketches the possibility of a general secularly justifiable language that can bind moral strangers. It does not indicate how moral strangers will in general be motivated to resolve issues peaceably, that is, in terms of such a language. There will always be those of passionate and particular conviction who will not be interested in this general secular language of peaceable collaboration among moral strangers. Such individuals will not enter into philosophical or political dialogue towards the goal of peaceable collaboration and therefore may be the subject of punitive and defensive force by secular governments who can justify themselves in terms of the general morality of peaceable moral strangers. This circumstance does not undermine the significance of particular belief. For example, the author is a believer.

References

1. Ayer AJ. Language, Truth, and Logic. Peter Smith: London; 1935.
2. Baynes K, Bohman J, McCarthy T (eds). After Philosophy. MIT Press: Cambridge, Mass; 1987.
3. Emanuel L, Emanuel EJ. The medical directive. JAMA, 1989; 261 (June 9): 3288–93.
4. Engelhardt HT, Jr. The Foundations of Bioethics. Oxford University Press; New York; 1986.
5. Engelhardt HT, Jr., Caplan A. (eds). Scientific Controversies. Cambridge University Press: Cambridge; 1987.
6. Engelhardt HT, Jr. Applied philosophy in the post-modern age: An augury. Journal of Social Philosophy 1989; 20 (June 2): 42–8.
7. Engelhardt HT, Jr. Bioethics and Secular Humanism: The Search for a Common Morality. Trinity Press International: Philadelphia; 1991.
8. Feshbach M. Health in the USSR: Organization, trends, and ethics. In Sass H-M, Massey RU (eds): Health Care System. Kluwer Academic Publishers: Dordrecht 1988; pp. 117–32.
9. Lyotard J-F. The Postmodern Condition, trans. Bennington G, Massumi B. Manchester University Press: Manchester; 1984.
10. MacIntyre A. After Virtue. Notre Dame University Press: Notre Dame, Indiana; 1981.
11. MacIntyre A. Whose Justice? Which Rationality? Notre Dame University Press: Notre Dame, Indiana; 1988.
12. MacIntyre A. Three Rival Versions of Moral Enquiry. Notre Dame University Press: Notre Dame, Indiana; 1990.
13. Rorty R. Contingency, Irony, and Solidarity. Cambridge University Press: New York; 1989.
14. Stevenson C. Facts and Values: Studies in Ethical Analysis. Greenwood Press: Westport, Connecticut; 1975.

2. Theories of justice

LARRY R. CHURCHILL

This chapter is a description of some of the major theories of justice, along with the implications of these theories for problems of resource allocation in medicine. The role of physicians in these decisions will also be discussed.

It is important to be clear about what part theory plays in ethical judgments, and why we should concern ourselves with theory. Why, after all, have a theory of justice? Will our ethical reasoning about resource allocation be shallow without theoretical sponsorship, or worse, our actions wrong?

The first part of this essay deals with the uses and role of theory, including what we can and cannot expect theory to do for us. The second part is a description of some of the major theories of justice which could be employed in allocation policies and decisions. While it is customarily thought that physicians must be exempt from considerations of justice in the treatment of individual patients, I will argue that the ethics of individual acts and practices cannot finally be separated from the concerns of just policy.

I. The role and uses of theory

Ethics is concerned with action, but not solely or simply with action. Ethics focuses on action *and* explanation, decisions *and* justification for those decisions. Ethics is not just what we do but what we do, and *why*.

The birth of theory in ethics can be allegorically stated as something like this.[1] It was that occasion when the son or daughter refused simply to accept the teachings of the parent just because they were the teachings of the parent, and insisted on some other grounds for their validity. When the child insisted not merely on assertion, but on argument, theory was added to morality and ethics was born. And we have been arguing ever since.

Sons and daughters question the authority of their elders because they encounter other ways of doing things, over the hills, in the next valley, in California, or the Netherlands. The elementary experience of comparison induces the need for *theory* as explicit, formalized and argued positions. In the Netherlands physicians practice euthanasia under carefully circumscribed conditions. Should we be doing

21

C. M. Kjellstrand and J. B. Dossetor (eds): Ethical Problems in Dialysis and Transplantation, 21–34.
© 1992 Kluwer Academic Publishers. Printed in the Netherlands.

the same in the United States, or if we are, should we do so explicitly rather than covertly? Oregon is working to prioritize the health needs of its Medicaid population. Should New York do the same? The British rarely offer hemodialysis to those over age 55. Would the U.S. health care system be better if we did likewise? Comparisons breed the need for theory, for rationales, justifications, for answers to the *why* question.

We are, of course, driven to theory in ethics by reasons other than those suggested in the allegory of origins. We also have recourse to theory when we sense our moral intuitions are inadequate, or at worst, bankrupt. Medical students, for example, when they encounter an abusive patient, or a patient dying from AIDS, may feel that the norms they have unself-consciously relied upon to guide them may not stretch to cover this situation. Beyond the encounter with differences and comparisons is the encounter with novelty, usually of a troubling sort.

Another less stressful kind of impetus to theory is the drive for higher levels of coherence. This is not simply the philosopher's drive, but a more general human need that seeks coherence in ethics among actions and principles, between persons, within lifetimes and across societies – a more comprehensive frame of reference to see how it all fits together, if it does. The sense that somehow it *should* all fit, or that we can at least see why it won't, is a basic human urge that gives occasion to theory.

So ethics is not just incidentally concerned with what is theoretically correct. What we think we 'ought' to do has no moral weight at all unless we get into theory. All persons are moral in the sense of being moved by 'oughts,' but not all are ethical, in the sense of employing critical self-conscious reflection on their moral hunches and intuitions.

The allegory about the origins of ethics, the birth of moral theory, also bespeaks the need of every generation to both rediscover and to invent theoretical constructs for itself. Medicine is best defining and sustaining itself when, for example, it is debating the Baby Doe regulations, or whether to join in preparation for nuclear war, or participate in capital punishment, or prepaid, gatekeeper health financing schemes. Medicine is most threatened as a profession when it allows these debates to be settled in nonmoral terms, such as those of economic, or legal constraints, or even when it allows the moral debate on such issues to exclude the values intrinsic to medical practice. None of these debates can dispense with theory. Medicine will be dead as a profession when it stops asking the 'why' question, when its ethic, including its sense of justice in allocation, ceases to be theoretical.

Theorizing is one way an ethical tradition generates its own resources for renewal. Those who believe they can dispense with theory are working with an unexamined theory, usually an intuitive, pragmatist theory – doing what just naturally seems right and what works, and effortless osmosis of moral truth. Being clear about what theories we are working with is an essential part of ethics.

A. *What theory cannot do: problem-solving*

It is widely thought that ethical theories can solve moral quandaries. For example, Bernard Gert ([3], p. 738) says, '...a normative ethical theory is an attempt to provide a systematic account of morality such that one will be able, at least in principle, to determine correct answers to at least some moral problems.' John Arras and Nancy Rhoden ([6], p. 6) make a similar claim in the Introduction to their anthology. 'It is our contention that, if answers to ethical issues are to be found, they will be found through the development of a cogent and comprehensive ethical theory – a theory that will both explain the principles of morality and give us a guide to their application.' Following this logic, the reason for having a theory of justice is that it would help us resolve quandaries of allocation. Physicians or policy-makers, then, faced with scarce resources, could make sound choices by *applying* the theory to the concrete issue before them.

This view of theory as a problem-solving apparatus may appear so evident that to challenge it will seem bizarre. Yet this view is at least misleading and I think actually false, for it strives to make theory do something it cannot do. Theories don't solve problems; persons solve problems. Gert, Arras and Rhoden offer a view of theory which gives it preeminence over the other aspects of ethics, such as judgment, perception and the insights of practice. The view of ethics which makes theory the final arbiter of moral problems is the view I want to challenge.

The typical view of how theory can solve problems is roughly this. Physicians in the course of their practice encounter *problems*, which are referred to *rules*, or *principles*, the rules or principles usually lead in different directions and so must be explored for cogence, given an order, and conflicts among them finally adjudicated by recourse to *theory*. And it is at this level of theory that the problem reaches resolution, for from the theoretical overview, a principle is endorsed and a best course of action is chosen and legitimated. The approach is 'bottoms-up,' then 'tops-down'. The articulation of the problem goes from the concrete to the abstract, from the particular to the universal, while the solution goes from abstract to the concrete, from the universal to its particular application. The real business of ethics, so this view says, occurs at the metalevel – in terms of contesting theories, Kant vs. Mill, Christianity vs. Marxism, libertarianism vs. paternalism, and so on. The contest of 'isms' occurs at a remove from the actual experiences of doctors, patients and families. This 'looking for answers in theories,' a vertical problem-solving, is what I want to argue against.

Assigning the problem-solving task to theory makes us overlook the way *persons* using theory (and other human skills) solve problems. Thus, we confuse a tool (ethical theory) with the skillful use of that tool. Theories don't yield answers, moral agents use theories to strive for an answer. But theories don't do the striving for them. The process is not automatic and there are lots of ways it goes wrong.

Moral agents with brilliant and subtle theories botch up their choices, just as I could possess a Stradivarius and play it poorly, or own a Lamborgini and still drive it like a Chrysler. Likewise elegant egalitarian, contract theories, cannot be simply applied to issues of justice in health care, much less to fairness in allocating the rescue machinery of hemodialysis.

The view of ethical theories as axioms in a deduction problem-solving process also reflects an enfeebled moral psychology. Answers to problems become standard mechanical products of theoretical prowess, not decisions reached in unique and personal ways by the particular people involved. G. Scott Davis ([2], p. 487) rightly claims that this is not only an implausible picture of moral agency, but perverse, as though we were looking at generic brand answers. In fact, each of us as moral actors puts our unique stamp on the decisions we make. Our moral decisions bear our mark, Davis says, just as 'pots belong to the potter', or sutures to the surgeon. As Aristotle would say, we are particularized moral craftsmen, not assembly-line conduits for 'cookie-cutter' answers. And this particularity is just as evident in devising good policy as it is in reaching good individual patient-care choices.

In a less direct and regulatory way theory does, of course, help in problem resolution. Just how this works, however, cannot be easily described and cannot be streamlined into a deductive paradigm. When wrestling with some practical dilemma we often seek to see the problem from some hypothetical vantage-point. We ask questions which *presume* the relevance of theoretical structures. For example, 'How should health outcomes weigh in distribution of health care resources?'; 'Is there a role for meritorious health behaviors in distributing benefits and burdens in health care?'; or 'What should be the place of age in considering eligibility for treatment of ESRD?,' and so on. These, and a wide variety of other maneuvers, are designed to clarify options, elicit assumptions and evoke hidden aspects of choices, and each could easily be referenced to and tested by one or more theories in ethics, for example, Kantian theory which stresses universalizability, utilitarianism which stresses calculations of greatest happiness, and so on.

Reflection on the dynamic of problem-solving indicates that we seek theoretical structures to illumine and often to justify our choices, but also that our choices about which theories are relevant is dependent on the problem at hand. There is a reflective oscillation between theory and practice, between the ideal conditions, stipulations and defining power of theory, on the one hand, and the actual circumstances of choice on the other. Between these stands the moral agent, in the place of judgment.

My claim is not that theory is irrelevant to problem-solving. Far from it. Only that theories do not solve problems and the idea that they give us some final court of appeals for our choices belies both the complexity of our experience and the role of judgment. Finally, of course, assigning the problem-solving task to theory in a unilateral way oversimplifies and warps theory as well.

B. *What theory cannot do: foundations*

It is sometimes asserted that a theory of justice is needed – not to solve problems – but to provide 'foundations' for our decisions. Without foundations, we are told, right and wrong judgments can be only antecdotal – referenced only to the particulars of cases, or the provincial norms of medical traditions. Robert Veatch, for example, in the 'Introduction' to A Theory of Medical Ethics, ([13], p. 5) says that the existing collection of codes and principles which physicians have devised is nothing more than 'a series of unsystematic, unreflective ethical stances or traditions.' He refuses to call these 'theories' but reserves that appellation to 'some more systematic structuring'.

Veatch, like many other philosophers, believes that theory is essential because it elucidates first principles. These first principles constitute the foundations on which sound judgments can rest.

Veatch is quite right to criticize the unthinking acceptance of moral custom in medicine as a theory of medical ethics. Yet what we should expect to replace custom is not a foundational truth, a sure grounding in universal first principles, but simply *critical reflection*. Theorizing does not need a lot of heavy logical or epistemological apparatus to get it going. All that is required is a willingness to suspend custom long enough to question it. Theorizing may, to be sure, result in a theory, that is, a set of rationales, reasons and supporting positions which are systematically linked. But the history of Western philosophy is full of the wreckage which ensues when such a structure is moved across situations, times and persons and claims to be *the* structure. We need not one theory of medical ethics, or one theory of justice, but many. But most of all we need an emphasis on *theorizing* as critical reflection rather than as securing foundations. It takes very little to launch theorizing – a variety of experiences to give comparisons, or minimally a supple enough imagination to realize that things could be otherwise.

'Theory' can elucidate the 'foundations' for moral choices if we take a more modest sense of both these terms.[2] If by 'theory' we mean, simply, critical reflection on moral practice, and if by 'foundations' we mean, simply the best reasons we can give, the most sense and coherence we can muster for our choices, then theory can and does reveal foundations. Probing for foundations is seeking to display more of the larger context in which particular choices take on the moral significance they have. Finding foundations does not and cannot mean discovering *the* foundations for moral choices generally, or some axiomatic first principles from which choices can always and securely be made. There are none. There is, of course, shallow or deep probing and better or worse reasoning for the particular choices of particular agents. The mistake is the wholesale effort to lay bare through theory the supporting structure for justice *once and for all*. This has been tried often enough that we should simply give it up as a bad idea and get on with the more pressing and important task of being conversant and critical about the choices before us.

II. Theories of justice and their relevance for the allocation of dialysis and transplantation

Since Aristotle 'justice' has been roughly formulated as giving each person his or her due, that is, treating equals equally and unequals according to their inequalities. The debates in theories of justice are largely concerned with which inequalities are relevant. Distributive justice focuses on benefits and burdens and how they affect individuals, groups or classes of people. Theories of distributive justice in health care are, therefore, ways of formulating principles or rules for the allocation of benefits and burdens so that the *relevant* (and only the relevant) inequalities come into play.

Using theories of distributive justice in health care is difficult for two reasons. First there is a vast array of procedures and services that fall under the category 'health care,' from facelifts to inoculations, from wellness clinics to heart transplants. Second, access to health care is valued differently not only by different people, but by the same person at different times. Health care may not seem important if we perceive ourselves as well, but as essential if we believe we are ill. Because of these factors, it has proven easier to gain clarity and consensus on other goods and services. Color televisions, for example, are universally distributed by market forces, so that the relevant inequality is the ability to pay. Olympic medals, by contrast, are distributed by athletic prowess, where inequality is measured by performance (not medically or chemically enhanced), and race, age or social status are irrelevant inequalities. In most societies access to some degree of public education is offered to all, and native intelligence, social standing, etc., are considered irrelevant inequalities. Burdens are borne in proportionately equal terms though tax-based revenue systems. In each of these and many other areas, the knotty issues of distribution are generally settled, but in health care (at least in the US) the question of what counts as a relevant inequality is contested terrain. Each society must finally settle on a method for allocating dialysis and transplant services, though there is no reason to believe that the method chosen must be the same as that by which goods and services are generally allocated, or the same method used for other health care goods and services. For example, preventive services and treatment for hypertension could be distributed in one fashion, and dialysis in another. It is an open question whether a unitary set of principles can speak to health care as a whole.

An exhaustive, or even a representative historical account of the many theories of justice which might be relevant to health care generally, and allocation of dialysis and transplantation services specifically, would be too much to attempt. I will confine myself to the major modern theories of justice, that is, to those which are usually cited as providing a way to sort out the relevant inequalities in distribution. I will review these theories not as contributions of specific theorists, but in terms of types, giving representative thinkers for each type. My aim is not to argue for one theory over others, but to suggest that each has assets and liabilities and that the task is to learn to incorporate the merits of each while being aware of its blindspots.

A. *Egalitarianism*

Egalitarian theories emphasize similarities or equalities among persons. Such theories typically embrace notions of intrinsic worth, that is, those aspects of persons which are *not* instrumental to achieving some other good, but in terms of which persons are to be valued for their own sake. Egalitarian theories of health care distribution focus on the *need* for services as the basic criterion in allocation, rather than money, insurance, social class or other factors. These other factors are deemed irrelevant for access to health care. Egalitarian theories are supported by recognition not only of the equal intrinsic worth of persons, but by a common human vulnerability to disease, disability and death, by a common condition of inability to predict the timing or extent of our health care needs, and by the importance of health services, both for life and health, but also for dignity and self-respect. Michael Walzer ([14], p. 89) puts it this way.

> Were medical care a luxury, these discrepancies [in access to care] would not matter much; but as soon as medical care becomes a socially recognized need, and as soon as the community invests in its provision, they matter a great deal. For then deprivation is a double loss – to one's health and to one's social standing. Doctors and hospitals have become such massively important features of contemporary life that to be cut off from the help they provide is not only dangerous but also degrading.

Many egalitarian theorists believe the best approach comes from applying the principles of John Rawls to health care. Rawls ([12], pp. 302–3) contends that inequalities in the distribution of the primary goods of a society can be tolerated only if these inequalities are to everyone's advantage. Whether health care is a primary good is a contested notion. Norman Daniels' ([9], pp. 41–57) scheme for equitable distribution argues for a fair 'equality of opportunity' to 'species-typical normal functioning.' Some degree of health care is clearly part of the provision for opportunity to achieve normal functioning, and the liberties and goods that accrue from normal functioning.

Egalitarians frequently speak of health care as a right. For some this is a right of equal access to all that is available, which would include dialysis, transplantation and any other advances in treating ESRD which may be developed. Others see this right more modestly as a right to a decent, or basic minimum, which may or may not include dialysis and transplant services.

The typical strengths of egalitarian theories are the emphases on intrinsic worth, the high ideals which they hold out for us, and the descriptive accuracies concerning things humans hold (and suffer) in common. Egalitarian theories frequently resonate with religious traditions which eschew social worth judgments for allocation, and favor the poor and disenfranchised. In this respect egalitarianism is frequently, but not always, aligned with communitarian values, as well as with contract theories.

The weaknesses of egalitarian approaches are in part definitional and operational. What, after all, is a health care 'need' and *who* should define it? Our health needs seem to expand daily and our appetite for health, at least in the US, has yet to find a natural limit. Guaranteeing everyone a right to treatment for ESRD, as has been done in the US, may in fact be so costly as to deprive the populace of other basic needs, both medical and non-medical. Utilitarian and libertarian approaches involve additional critiques of egalitarianism and these will become evident as we proceed.

B. *Utilitarianism*

Utilitarian theories reference the rightness or wrongness of actions or policies to the good or bad consequences they generate. While egalitarian theories emphasize intrinsic worth, utilitarian approaches avoid judging policies by the intention of such policies and make judgments of rightness rest on the empirical results. Right acts and policies are those which issue in the most good achieved, or the greatest net happiness for the greatest number. For some utilitarians, such as Jeremy Bentham [7], all kinds of happiness count, so that the calculation of the greatest good is purely quantitative. Others, such as John Stuart Mill [10], have developed hierarchies of happiness such that the higher pleasures, or those distinctive to human fulfillment, will count for more.

Utilitarianism does not endorse, as is sometimes thought, egoistic hedonism, such that only my own pleasure counts in the calculations. Rather it is the well-being or happiness of all that matters, and each is to be counted neutrally and equally. If anything, utilitarian theories may actually require more disinterested judgments about our own lives than most of us are capable of.

Regarding health care, and dialysis and transplantation more precisely, utilitarian approaches ask us to weigh the benefits and burdens of various policies of allocation, and to be guided by the results. Would the greatest net happiness be achieved by policies which granted availability to all, or by policies which restrict access in some fashion, or which possibly dismantled the entire technological apparatus for treating ESRD? While utilitarians do not usually advocate radical positions of change, they are theoretically open to any actions which would achieve the desired end. In making such calculations for health care a great deal would have to be considered, for example, the happiness of those treated, the tax burdens of those who pay, the impact of discontinuing, curtailing or expanding a program, and so on. The well-being of patients, non-patients, physicians and others, indeed all others would be important. The key element here is the absence of intrinsic, or innate values which might countervail our ability to assess the outcomes, and the irrelevance of motives and intentions. Goodness, in utilitarian thinking, is not a state of will or an internal motivation of the heart, but a real, measurable item in the world. Moreover, it is not just what I want, but what would be good when the well-being of all is considered.

The strengths of utilitarian approaches are numerous. The emphasis on empirical reality rather than inner motives makes for more accessible and public judgments and can serve to open discussion to a broad range of participants. Additionally, utilitarianism, at least in its most influential forms, encourages objectivity in the sense that each person's happiness counts but no one's happiness counts more than others. Some are attracted to utilitarianism for its simplicity. Rather than a complex bevy of rules and maxims, a single principle referenced to outcomes and events is offered. Finally, utilitarian schemes seem to have a natural affinity with democratic governmental practices. It is no accident that Bentham's and Mill's utilitarian philosophies have underwritten a number of social and political reforms in England in the 19th and 20th centuries.

Still the liabilities are substantial. A standard for justice which is referenced solely to outcomes must rely on the ability to predict outcomes correctly. This can make for a difficult task. Others have worried that utilitarian approaches are counter-intuitive. If everyone's happiness is to be counted as equal to my own, does this mandate the most extraordinary self-sacrifice? Moreover, if everyone's happiness is to count equally, does this mean that the physician has equal obligations to her current ESRD patient and to a perfect stranger? Utilitarianism would seem to undercut some of our most deep-seated notions of loyalty and fidelity. Finally, and perhaps most importantly, does the emphasis on the greatest happiness mean that great suffering for a few can be tolerated so long as the vast majority benefit? Would this encourage neglect of patients to achieve the greater social good? Perhaps these questions indicate why no single theory of justice has gained universal acceptance in health care.

C. *Libertarianism*

Libertarian approaches to justice stand in stark contrast to the two previously discussed. Whereas both egalitarian and utilitarian approaches present alternative conceptions of the common good, libertarian thinking denies the existence of a common good altogether.

Robert Nozick ([11], pp. 32–33) states it forcefully. Pointing out that as individuals we frequently undergo sacrifices for a greater personal good, Nozick asks:

> Why not, similarly, hold that some persons have to bear some costs that benefit other persons more, for the sake of the overall social good? But there is no *social entity* with a good that undergoes some sacrifice for its own good. There are only individual people, different individual people, with their own individual lives. Using one of these people for the benefit of others, uses him and benefits the others. Nothing more.

Libertarianism, as the name suggests, values liberty, and the cardinal virtue is non-interference with others. This is not to say that other virtues – courage, loyalty, respect for others, beneficence – are not also valued, but only liberty is a *funda-*

mental right. The Bill of Rights of the US Constitution is frequently cited as a prominent example of libertarian thinking. The rights of free speech, assembly, religious worship and so on are seen primarily as rights to be left alone, rights not to be coerced by others, especially by government. Positive rights, rights that require obligations from others for their fulfillment, are not rights at all but claims which can only be satisfied by violating the basic rights of others. Hence, for libertarians there is no right to health care services, since this would involve coercing taxpayers to fund it and physicians to provide it. Inequities in health and health care are then seen as unfortunate, but not unfair. If the poor die from lack of dialysis or transplant services while others pay for it and survive, this may be regrettable, but it is not unjust. If charitable tendencies in society prevail such that doctors and hospitals give to the poor what they need, then they are to be commended. But there is no duty to provide it, and the poor have no claim to demand it.

Libertarian approaches place a high premium on protection of property, including financial resources. Possessions are seen as extensions of their owners. In a frequently quoted article against a right to health care, Robert Sade ([5], p. 1288) claims that since a physician owns his professional skills, he is entitled to do with them as he pleases. As bread belongs to the baker who made it, to dispose of as he wishes, so medical services belong to the physician. To force him into a fee schedule, to require him to provide services or to see patients he does not choose, is a fundamental breech of liberty.

Justice, in libertarian terms, is simply respecting the freedoms of persons and keeping hands off what they rightfully own. The idea that someone else may have a right to what one owns is frequently attributed, in libertarian thinking, to envy. Just because the poor envy the health care services of the rich does not entitle them to it. Rights claims, when they require redistribution of property, should be seen as nothing more than the politics of envy, so the libertarian argument often goes.

The strengths of libertarian thinking are obvious, at least to many Americans. The U.S. health care system is basically libertarian in orientation, distributing the goods and services of health care on the basis of purchasing power and the ownership of health insurance. Libertarian approaches dovetail with laissez faire economics, in health care and in most other sectors of society. In addition to its protection of economic freedoms, libertarianism appeals to our sense of respect for personal freedoms. This strikes a favourable cord with both patients and physicians. For patients it can mean the ability to choose one's doctor and negotiate the conditions of one's care. For physicians freedom to practice is often translated as freedom to make clinical judgments without interference and is seen, therefore, not merely as politically appropriate, but as the essence of professionalism, as 'good medicine.' Finally, libertarianism serves as a warning about the growth and hegemony of state power, and as such has a lasting appeal to anyone at all distrustful of concentration of power in whatever form.

The weaknesses of libertarian approaches are the strengths of egalitarian and utilitarian philosophies. First, libertarianism seems blind to commonalities among people, and the degree of shared life which is part of contemporary societies. In some of its more strident emphases on negative freedom, libertarian positions seem better suited to individuals attempting to break away from the repressive societies of the past. It isn't clear that the simple ethic of protecting freedoms is the best or only value for citizens of modern industrial democracies. Other critics have focused on the property rights orientation of libertarianism. Historically, it isn't always clear that current property holdings have been acquired fairly (by noncoercive means). Hence, some redistributive schemes which favor the less well off may amount to restorative justice. Additionally, portraits of physicians which view them as holding knowledge and skills as private possessions for sale ignore the large contributions from public funds which train physicians, support hospitals and subsidize the payment for patient services. Medicine could not be practiced in anything like its present form without the 'coercive' hand of government subsidies and public tax support. Finally, libertarian approaches ring true only if health is thought of as a private possession rather than a public good. A completely individual approach to health needs, in which concerted public and social approaches were eliminated, would result in a substantial diminishment of health status generally. This critique does not, to be sure, make the case for a broad right to health care services, or to dialysis or transplantation. Rather it shows that as valuable as libertian values may be in many realms of political life, it is not clear that freedom is a primary criterion for distributives justice in health care. Unequal possessions may not be the most relevant inequality for health care.

After this review of strengths and weaknesses of major theories it might be tempting to conclude that theorizing leads us nowhere. That conclusion would be too strong. The conclusion to draw is that no one theory will provide the answer and that our best approach is a pluralistic one, a reasoned approach which combines what is best and what is workable to the problems at hand.

III. Theories of justice and the role of physicians[3]

The physician's response to this examination of theories of justice may be less than enthusiastic. Many seem to feel that policy reforms are needed, but that this discussion of allocation should go on at a remove from clinical interactions. For some there is not only a separation of health policy questions from clinical decisions, but a positive moral obligation for physicians, *qua* clinical caregivers, to be disinterested in policy and allocation altogether. Norman Levinsky ([4], p. 1573) puts it this way. Physicians are 'required to do everything they believe may benefit each patient without regard to costs, or other societal considerations.' The problem is perceived as one of divided loyalties and is to resolved by choosing always for the patient.

Robert Veatch ([13], p. 15 ff) believes this view of medical ethics constitutes 'the Hippocratic tradition,' which, he says 'mandates that the physician do what he or she thinks is in the patient's interest, and does not recognize a qualification such as 'unless the costs are great in comparison to the benefits to be gained,' or take into account what economists call "alternative costs"...' Veatch's own reformulation of medical ethics retains the individualized ethic he finds in the 'Hippocratic tradition,' and he calls for practitioners to be 'exempt from the general moral requirements of the principles of justice' ([13] p. 330) insofar as they are involved in relationships with patients. This reading of medical ethics is not inimical to policy *per se*, or the physician as a policy-maker. Rather it holds that policies and patient care obligations are and must be, distinct and separate.

Part of the force and staying power of this view is practical. Physicians in the US who do attempt to be responsive to cost and distributional problems cannot be assured that following just policies or reasonable procedures in treating individual patients will result in a greater good. While US physicians directly control roughly 80% of all health care resources, they have no assurances that dollars saved by judicious restraint with one patient will benefit that same patient at a later time, or other patients with greater needs or more malleable diseases. Hence there is no incentive for individual physicians to say 'No' to marginal care for their patients. In the absence of a societal mandate and an organized system of distribution, every 'No' seems ad hoc and arbitrary. Decisions of physicians to withhold even the most marginal treatments occur in the absence of a shared fiscal and moral context. As Norman Daniels ([1], p. 1383) says of our system of health care financing and distribution, 'It is not closed under constraints of justice.'

Compounding the problem still further is the contemporary emphasis on patient autonomy. The impact of individual patient choices upon the distribution of health care resources has been considered irrelevant. The right to self-determination was first used as a justification for refusal of treatment, and perhaps because of this there was no initial conflict between an individual patient's wishes and a fair distribution of resources. However, it is becoming increasingly evident that individual choices dramatically affect the resources available for others.

The tradition of patient advocacy in medical ethics, the practical difficulties of realizing patient-care gains from restraint, and the contemporary emphasis on patient autonomy conspire to remove considerations of justice from clinical encounters. This is, in part, as it should be. The image of clinicians rationing in an ad hoc fashion at the bedside, on a purely case-by-case basis, inventing policy as the occasions arises, is most unsavory. Yet this image may have such an arresting and repugnant power that we fail to consider that physicians will inevitably need to make some 'policy' decisions in the course of caring for patients. Ethical concerns about the fair distribution of health care resources cannot remain detached from the ethic of individual patient care. Total fidelity to the patient before one and a 'hang the costs' attitude is itself a policy.

It is both wise and necessary that policy decisions at the macrolevel guide the general distribution of resources. Ethical decisions about the availability of dialysis and transplantation, for example, will depend on a wide variety of factors which are ultimately social decisions about the proper use of resources within a competing list of health needs. And on an even larger social level, health needs generally compete with support for education, defense, the arts, and on and on. All societies must ask about the importance of transplanting kidneys rather than building intensive care units or providing extensive prenatal care. All societies must decide how many surgeons it will seek to train,what new cyclosporines it will test, whether kidney donor policies should be voluntary or assumptive, etc. Yet no policies, however well-conceived or definitive, can cover the diverse range of choices involved in caring for seriously ill persons. Even the best and most thorough policies will not relieve the physician and the patient of all choices. Moreover, and more importantly, no policy-level decision will be feasible without the concurrence of physicians and patients who see the wisdom of such policies and are morally motivated to live within them.

The detachment of theories of justice from particular clinical choices cannot be sustained in a world in which health care is seen as a requirement for a minimally decent life, and in which so much of the good for humankind has been laid at medicine's door. We can argue that health care is overvalued and work to de-mythologize it and loosen its hold on our sense of well-being. Callahan [8] has argued that some re-ordering of our priorities is sorely needed. Until this reformation in attitudes and values occurs, physicians cannot remove themselves from the issues of just policy or make themselves immune to its influence. What is required is a more integrated ethical framework, one that puts individual patient care questions and social justice questions simultaneously into focus. Such a framework will allow us to look at individual patient treatment decisions and at problems of distribution at the same time. This does not mean that patient advocacy must be abandoned, or even displaced as the cardinal principle of medical ethics. Rather it means that we can no longer pretend to make individual decisions in a social vacuum. Issues of justice and theories of justice will always be present, if not always visible, as a factor in patient care. Every clinical encounter is to some extent the result of a policy, even if only the result of a lack of an explicit policy, for we express our values both by what we seek to achieve through regulation and by what we seek to achieve through its absence.

Notes

1. For this allegory I am indebted to Professor Ruel W. Tyson, Jr., who attributes it to the late Professor Leo Strauss.
2. For an interesting and original work on 'theory' see Annette Baier's *Postures of the Mind* (University of Minnesota Press, 1985), especially chapters 11 and 12. For a critique of foundational thinking, see Richard Rorty's *Consequence of Pragmatism* (University of Minnesota Press, 1982), and *Contingency, Irony and Solidarity* (Cambridge University Press, 1989). Elizabeth Wolgast (*The Grammar of Justice*, Cornell University Press, 1987) takes a Wittgensteinian approach. She argues that 'The question, raised so often by moral philosophers, as to the real foundation of morality asks

for something impossible – that we supply a foundation for morality as if it were *not* part and parcel of our lives and the process of learning our language' (p. 212). I am indebted to these and other like-minded philosophers for the approach I take here.
3. The ideas in this section receive a more extensive discussion focused on intensive care situations in Marion Danis and Larry R. Churchill, Autonomy and the Commonwealth, *The Hastings Center Report* (Jan./Feb., 1991).

References

1. Daniels N. Why saying no to patients in the United States is so hard. New Engl J Med 1986; 314: 1380–3.
2. Davis GS. Warcraft and the fragility of virtue. Soundings 1987; LXX: 475–94.
3. Gert B. Ethics: Objectivism in ethics. In Reich W(ed): The Encyclopedia of Bioethics 1. Macmillian: New York, New York 1978.
4. Levinsky N. The doctor's master. New Engl J Med 1984; 311: 1573–5.
5. Sade R. Medical care as a right: A refutation. New Engl J Med 1971; 285: 1288 ff.
6. Arras J. Rhoden N. Ethical issues in modern medicine, third edition. Mayfield Publishing Company: Palo Alto, California; 1989.
7. Bentham J. An introduction to the principles of morals and legislation. Penguin Books: New York, New York; 1987 (1789).
8. Callahan D. What kind of life. Simon and Schuster: New York, New York; 1990.
9. Daniels N. Just health care. Cambridge University Press: Cambridge, England; 1985.
10. Mill JS. Utilitarianism. Penguin Books: New York, New York; 1987 (1861).
11. Nozick R. Anarchy, state and utopia. Basic Books: New York, New York; 1974.
12. Rawls J. A theory of justice. Harvard University Press: Cambridge, Mass; 1971.
13. Veatch RM. A theory of medical ethics. Basic Books: New York, New York; 1981.
14. Walzer M. Spheres of justice: A defense of pluralism and equality. Basic Books: New York, New York; 1983.

PART TWO

Selection and commercialization

3. Ethics issues in selection for dialysis and transplantation: the duty of advocacy

JOHN B. DOSSETOR & CARL M. KJELLSTRAND

Chronic dialysis and transplantation highlight a number of ethical issues in medicine in an unprecedented way. The issues and outcome are clear: if a patient is accepted to dialysis his life can be prolonged for decades, if not he will certainly die. Analyses and reviews, some of which appear elsewhere in this book clearly indicate that sex, race, economic circumstances and even politics may influence who receives treatment and who dies. Thus. the physician's fulfilment of his duty to justice is starkly apparent and failure to meet it appears to be common. The curves for acceptance to dialysis rise steeply everywhere suggesting that rationing still goes on and that nowhere are all needy patients being accepted for treatment. How does one solve this problem?

The only limit is economic. If enough money were available enough machines could be bought and staff trained so that everyone was treated. But since this is not the case, how should one select patients for treatment when not all can be treated? Each dialysis machine can only treat 4 or 6 patients. Young patients can live three and four decades, older patients may be dead within 5 years of the start of dialysis. Is a 30 year old patient who takes up 30 years of machine time worth eight 75 year old patients who each take up only 5 years of machine time?

Transplantation offers an equally stark choice. Most people see transplantation as vastly improving their quality of life, but who is to receive it? Again, age sex and economic power seem to dictate the distribution of organs. Unlike dialysis machines, Governments cannot make or buy cadaveric kidneys so everyone depends on the goodwill of the public. Yet the rising transplant rate has faltered. Why is this? Is it evidence of distrust by the public of Government or of a 'medical system' which may be perceived as taking from the masses and giving to the powerful? To what degree do dialysis physicians, with vested interests in having 'good candidates' for dialysis, prevent such patients from fulfilling their equally valid role as ideal candidates for transplantation? Does every dialysis physician have an obligation to work for procurement of more transplantable kidneys?

This chapter will address these ethical issues in selection by using the schematic outline shown in Figure 1. The figure shows the wide range of issues involved. The main areas are:

C. M. Kjellstrand and J. B. Dossetor (eds): Ethical Problems in Dialysis and Transplantation, 37–52.
© 1992 *Kluwer Academic Publishers. Printed in the Netherlands.*

38

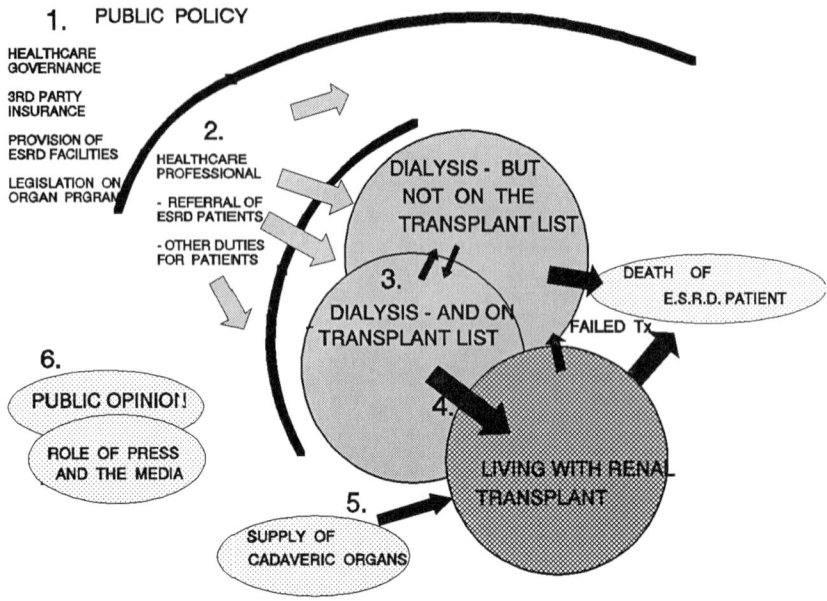

Figure 1. Diagram of interactions in chronic renal failure.

1. public policy concerning dialysis and transplantation;
2. the role of healthcare professionals and the efficacy of referral systems by which ESRD patients gain access to treatment;
3. the policies and criteria which dictate the form of dialysis offered to each patient and for placement on the transplant waiting list;
4. the criteria for selection from those on the transplant waiting list when an organ becomes available;
5. the adequacy of measures in place for organ procurement from cadaveric sources; and
6. the role played by the press and the media in informing public opinion. Public opinion is the final arbiter of the whole system both in theory and, ultimately, in fact.

Although these areas will be systematically treated, they are intimately related and should not be seen as separate except for discussion purposes. Thus, in a given constituency, where public policies are conservative, budget constraints very tight, and nephrologists in private fee-for-service practice, one might conjecture finding a restrictive ESRD referral policy per million population (pmp) especially limiting referral of elderly patients or those with concurrent disease, together with views that transplantation as a treatment modality has limited value, and lack of enthusiasm for cadaveric organ procurement. Conversely, in another constituency, where one may suppose that public policy supports a generous ESRD agenda but where nephrologists are on salary, one might expect to see a high rate of ESRD referral pmp with widely available options for dialysis, especially at home, together with a high transplantation rate and an efficient government supported organ procurement policy. These two examples are fictitious, but attempt to illustrate how factors affecting these six areas can work in various ways to shape treatment. Similar inter-dependency of different ESRD functions becomes evident, below, in discussion of the 'chances of being transplanted'.

There can be no doubt that there is much variation in different countries in the West. To compare some of them we have tabulated (see Table 1) data from various sources for 1988 [1–4] on: a) the incidence of ESRD pmp, b) the rate of transplan-tation pmp, c) the prevalence of ESRD pmp, overall, d) the prevalence of ESRD patients on dialysis and e) the prevalence of ESRD patients with renal transplants. We have compared 11 countries selected quite arbitrarily. From them, further cal-culations have been made of the 'chances for an ESRD patient of being trans-planted' in different countries, using two methods.

I. The incidence of ESRD

Figure 2 (taller bars) shows the incidence of new cases of ESRD per million popu-lation (pmp) for 1988, for the 11 arbitrarily selected countries. It varies from 34 pmp/yr (Ireland) to 144 pmp/yr (USA). No one knows, of course, the actual annual incidence of chronic renal failure in Western countries but an educated guess might

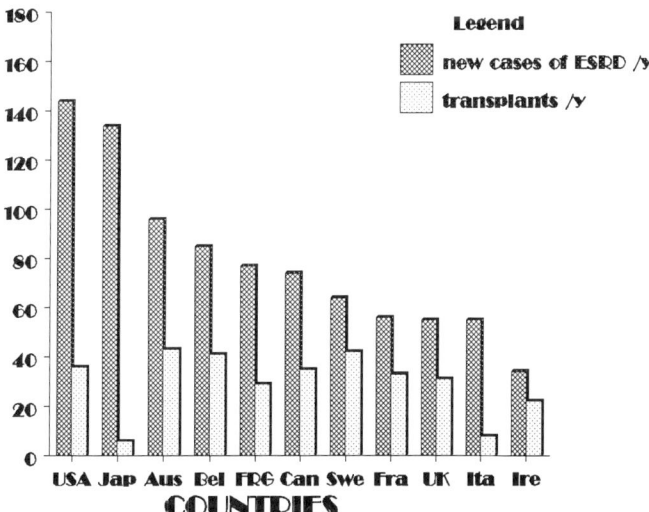

Figure 2. Incidence of ESRD and of renal transplants in different countries, 1988.

be in the range of 80–110 patients pump. This guess does not rule out the possibility that renal failure is much commoner in the USA and Japan than in Ireland but the data permits speculation that the selection criteria might also contribute significantly to the difference. To take these speculations further one would need the incidence further broken down by sex, age group, diagnostic group, concurrent disease, and race.

II. The prevalence of ESRD: overall, and in its two treatment modalities

Figure 3 shows the prevalence of ESRD patients in 1988 for the 11 arbitrarily selected countries, as well as the numbers who were being maintained on dialysis or living because of a transplant. The overall prevalence varies from 226 pmp (Ireland) to 778 pmp (Japan), and the % of these who had been transplanted varies from 61% (Ireland) to 18% (Italy) and 7% in Japan.

What would the prevalence level off at if programs captured all patients with ESRD at all ages and had time to come into dynamic equilibrium with deaths? No one knows, of course, but it would certainly be much higher than 500 ESRD patients pmp – and might well be as high as 1000–1200 pmp. This notion receives support from the evidence which relates prevalence of ESRD treatment to national income as measured by per capita gross national product (see Figure 4). There is a correlation coefficient of 0.87 for this data from 35 countries [5], establishing the fact – though close examination of the data reveals interesting national differences.

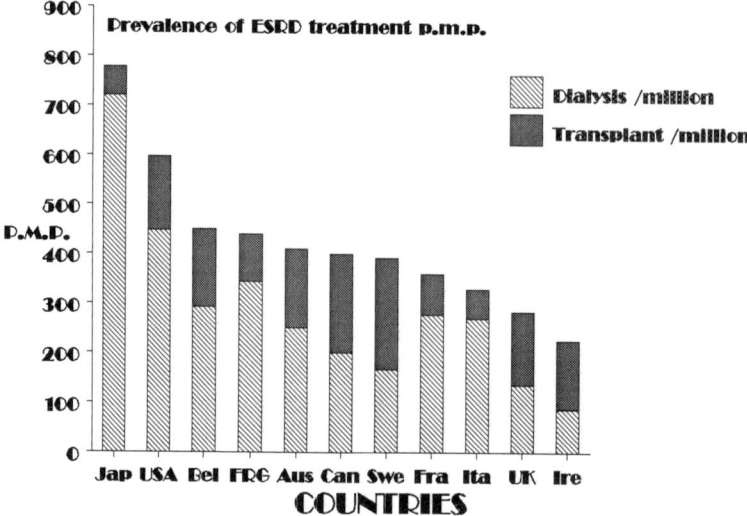

Figure 3. Dialysis and transplantation in context of ESRD treatment.

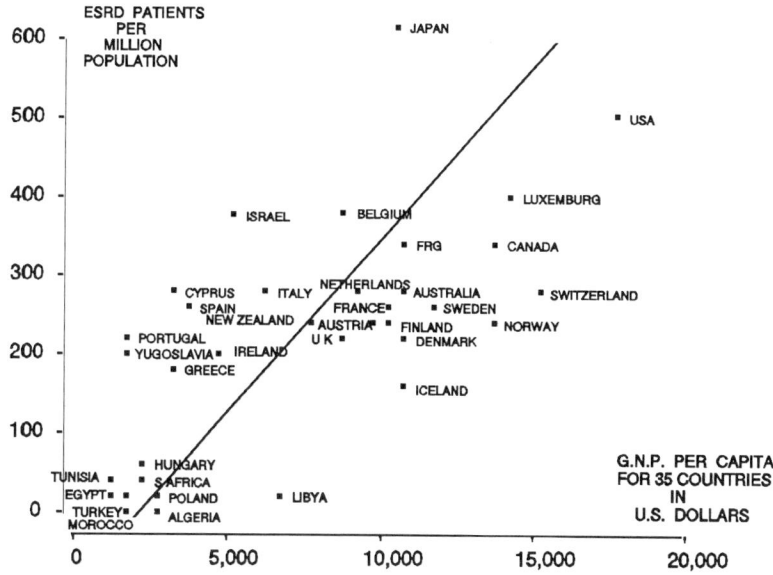

Figure 4. Prevalence of ESRD treatment per million population plotted against national income as GNP per capita (EDTA data).

III. The transplantation rate and transplantation chance

Figure 2 (lower bars) shows the transplant rate for 1988 for the 11 selected countries. The rate is above 40 pmp only in Austria, Belgium and Sweden and is lowest in Japan (6 pmp) and Italy (8 pmp).

The data permit one to calculate the 'chances of being transplanted' in a given year by two methods, as shown in Figure 5. Method a) is the annual transplant rate as a percentage of the annual incidence of ESRD. Method b) uses the transplant rate in relation to the prevalence of ESRD on dialysis, but also *makes an arbitrary assumption than only 33% of the dialysis pool is on the transplant waiting list.* It so happens that both methods give a comparable estimate of the 'chances of being transplanted' which varies from 5% in Japan and 12% in Italy to 50% in Canada and approximately 66% in Sweden, U.K. and the Republic of Ireland. However it is important not to fool oneself when thinking about the transplant chance! Thus a low transplant chance by method a) may reflect a low transplant rate, or a proportionately high acceptance rate with a normal transplant rate; and a low transplant chance by method b) may reflect a low transplant rate; or a proportionately high dialysis population (prevalence) in association with a normal transplant rate. In like

42

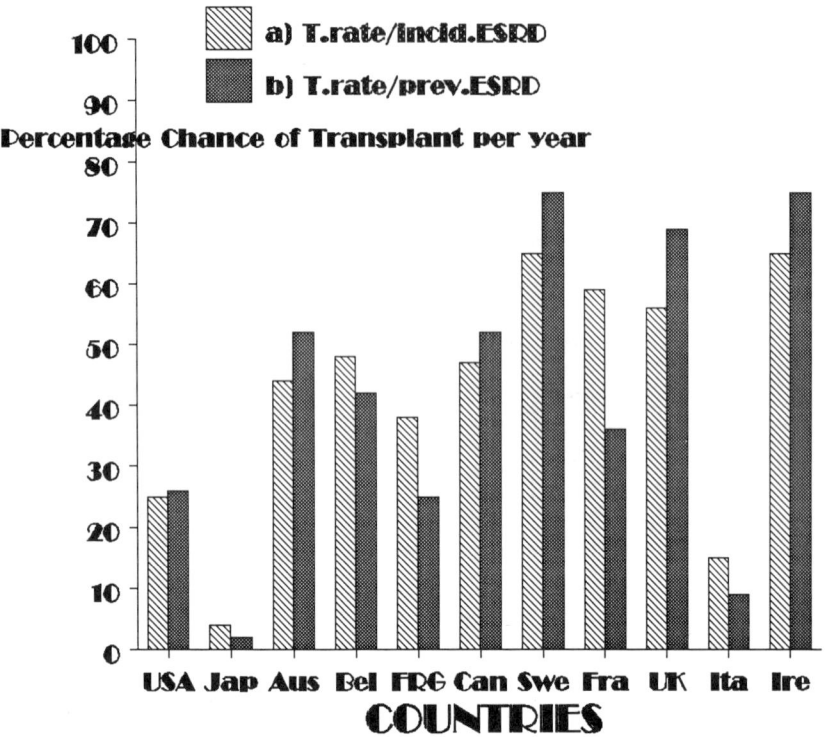

Figure 5. Chances of being transplanted in different countries in 1988. 2 methods of calculation (see text).

manner, there are several different ways of interpreting a high transplant chance – for example in the Republic of Ireland. The transplant chance reflects ones chances of transplantation after acceptance for ESRD treatment. But, the low 'chances' for patients in USA and Japan are mainly due to their very high acceptance rates, the two highest in the world.

IV. The ethical issues in selection

The ethics issues inhere to the dynamic equilibrium which one can assume to be present in each of these jurisdictions. Are they working towards that level of dynamic equilibrium what is dictated by public policy? Are there aspects which are unjust to ESRD patients? If so, what other data would be required to pin down such speculation? By what standards can any of these equilibria be judged to be just or unjust?

A. *Public policy*

Broadly speaking, all 11 countries have legislation which entitles all citizens to adequate treatment of ESRD. In the USA, for example, specific legislation was passed which entitled ESRD patients under 65 to treatment under at federal government expense, even though those who could not afford third part insurance (15% of the population) would not be covered for other diseases. Patients aged 65 years or more were already covered under Medicare regulations.

While it often appears that there may be rationing of entitlement for certain sections of the population, it is by no means easy to determine why this might be so. Whereas government is the arbiter of how much money to put into facilities for treatment, great freedom is granted to the medical profession to act as gate-keepers for entry into specific programs, in addition to their specific ethical obligations to be advocates for those with specific conditions. Thus, referral practices rather than public policy is more likely to reveal ethical problems, in the various systems in different countries. This is especially so if one supposes that the data quoted above represent a dynamic equilibrium for which the nephrologists have considerable ethical responsibility.

B. *The role of physicians and other healthcare professionals in ESRD referral*

The ethical obligations that physicians owe patients have generally been described under 'justice, beneficence, non-maleficence and respect for autonomy'. Under beneficence, we wish particularly to stress the *duty of advocacy*. Indeed, it might be singled out as a fifth principle.

By this we mean the obligation of physicians not only to be advocates for *individual* patient's needs but also for *groups* of patients. Physicians have a duty to be educators of the public and of colleagues about the benefits that their treatment can give. If a general practitioner does not understand that 70 year old patients may live happy, active and meaningful lives on dialysis they will not refer them. Nephrologists cannot escape responsibility for this. They should advocate their referral.

There is also the obligation to put pressure on bureaucracies and government to supply the needed equipment, competing with other healthcare specialities as well as non-health systems, such as education. In the 'best of all worlds', where a reasoned approach is possible towards unlimited public funds, calm discussion would solve such dilemmas, letting the facts speak for themselves. However, such a state of affairs is, and will remain, a distant dream. Fiscal constraints will always drive us back to QALYs and the like. Physicians must compete as advocates for their patients, pressing their patients' case in the forum of public opinion, and making sure that the older patient is not sacrificed on the altar of cost effectiveness. There is nothing efficient about serious illness; and ESRD brings down all groups and strata in society.

Broadly speaking, the factors which operate to limit free access for ESRD treatment are:

(a) Non-referral by family physicians
(b) Nephrologists misconceiving the utility of treatment
  i. systemic disease causing ESRD: SLE, diabetes mellitus
  ii. concurrent serious disease not causing ESRD: neoplastic disease, atherosclerosis and its complications, coronary heart disease, mental handicap, etc.
  iii. age
  iv. discrimination (often subconsciously) on grounds of gender, language, race, remoteness of domicile, and supposed lack of compliance.

Factors a) and b) are very difficult to distinguish from each other. Who provides the data on which family physicians form their referral patterns if it is not the specialists in nephrology? It does not seem possible to separate cause and effect, in such situations.

The situation in the U.K. is reviewed in this volume by Wing, who has previously noted the effect which government limitation of in-hospital dialysis facilities had on the development of ESRD treatment in that country [6]. It was noted that there was a smaller proportion of patients on dialysis over the age of 65 years in the United Kingdom than in other countries, which still persists. The nephrologists claimed that they placed every patient who was referred to them, with few exceptions, onto dialysis and did not believe that they might be responsible for what looked like an example of age discrimination. It was true that there were government restrictions on the number of dialysis units, but it was not thought that this was the primary cause. On further investigation, it became apparent that the cause was a perception on the part of referring physicians that there was no point in referring the older patients as they believed that they would not be accepted [7]. This belief, as it happened, was a false belief though there was a dearth of facilities, as Wing describes in Chapter 17.

A somewhat similar situation was evident with respect to ESRD in diabetic patients about 12 years ago. It was widely believed by diabetologists that dialysis units would not accept diabetic patients in CRF for treatment. This was so. It was believed by the nephrologists that such patients would develop gangrene in peripheral parts of the body if cannulae were inserted in atherosclerotic peripheral arteries, and that patients would all become blind after a year or so on hemodialysis (because of the need for repeated heparinization, etc). These largely unproven perceptions were, in fact, placed in the minds of diabetologists by nephrologists at a time when: i) all vascular access was in peripheral arteries, ii) before arteriovenous anastomoses became a common vascular access procedure, iii) before proximal arterial subcutaneous graft by-passes were developed, and iv) before chronic ambulatory peritoneal dialysis (CAPD) had become commonplace. The result of these

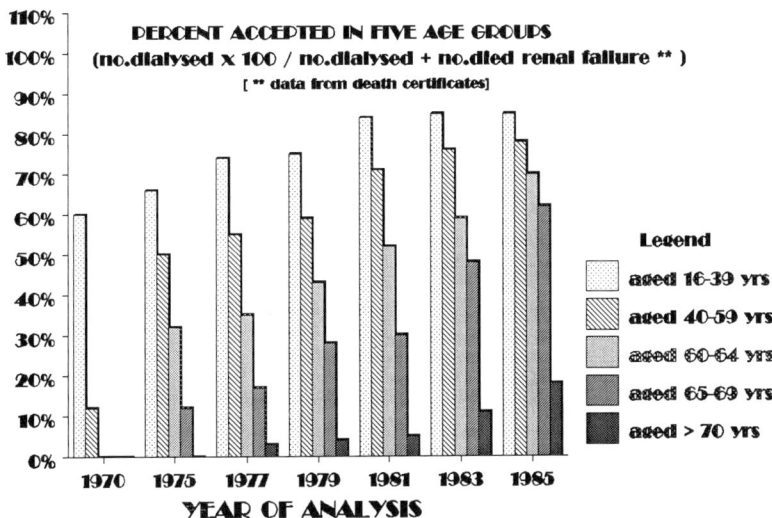

Figure 6. Changing acceptance of patients to dialysis with increasing age.

perceptions was that diabetologists stopped referring patients in renal failure throughout most of the 1960s and 1970s.

In that instance pioneer work in Minneapolis, in particular, showed that diabetic patients would do well on ESRD management, especially transplantation[8,9]. Even then it took about 5 years before the intake of diabetic patients with ESRD rose to its current plateau of 25% of all new ESRD patients [10].

It is evident that physician referral practices are critical to making the opportunity for dialysis available to patients, and there may be many physicians who still are slow to refer patients in the older age groups. Figure 6 shows the rates at which dialysis referrals, pmp/yr, for different age groups have been changing over time. The slope of referrals rises more slowly for the older decades (evidence of slower referral rates) even though it later increases to a higher level. The percentage referral is derived from the expression (no. dialysed in each age group × 100/[no. dialysed + death certificate evidence of renal death] for each age group). While admitting that death certificate evidence may be unreliable, it seems clear that there is probably no referral problem for younger age groups, but probably a referral problem does exist for the elderly.

Is there an ethical risk of 'over-dialysis'? It may be speculated that when the 'deep pocket' of government is paying for it patients may accept the offer of dialysis when it is not really in their best interests to do so. This would only apply to the very old, or those with lives which are severely burdened by physical or neurological handicap. Obviously, this is an ethical 'loaded' issue as judgment of 'best interests' can be very difficult and must always be decided on a case by case basis. Nevertheless, 'over-dialysis', if it occurs (and this has not been established) would be most likely to be found in situations where the dialysis unit is government funded and nephrologists are fee earning. Conversely, it is possible that when the unit is privately operated but government pays a dialysis fee, the mix of patients may become slanted towards young patients with better self-care habits and less concurrent disease, as these would seem to be more economic to look after on a fixed fee system [11]. Some aspects, as far as the USA is concerned, are touched in the Chapter 6 by Alan Hull, in this volume.

C. *Dialysis, or dialysis with a view to transplantation?*

The third set of ethical dilemmas concerns decisions on the mode of dialysis – CAPD, or hemodialysis (in-centre, assisted self-care, home hemodialysis, etc.) – and whether or not the patient is placed on the transplant waiting list.

Most centres believe they are giving each patient the treatment modality they most prefer. However, while making that claim, one must acknowledge that there are many variables operating on each patient's choice. Such variables include the academic and research interests of local nephrologists, the size of the unit, the balance between in-centre and home dialysis programs, the local nephrologists' interest in nephro-immunology and transplant immunology (in contrast to the skeletal, cerebral, atherosclerotic and other aspects of long term dialysis), and proximity to a transplantation unit. In many transplant units the thrust for HLA typing, cadaver kidney procurement and post transplant medical supervision has come from local nephrologists. Elsewhere, large dialysis units operate without close association with a transplant unit and deep commitment by nephrologists to transplantation is less likely.

Another important variable is the means by which both nephrologist and transplant physician are remunerated. In countries where dialysis physicians are not on salary, the key factor in nephrologists' income is the fee earned for each dialysis. This set of circumstances might temper, subconsciously at least, their enthusiasm for transplantation. The phenomenon termed 'trapping in dialysis' supposes that nephrologists subconsciously drift away from the transplant option, perceive that dialysis provides a safer way of life – if not as high a quality, for those who are successfully transplanted. This may prevent them from fully exploring transplantation as a treatment option for their patients, or making it as readily available as it might be.

The percentage of patients on transplant waiting lists in different countries might reflect differences in nephrologists' gatekeeper function, dependent on such factors as: belief that dialysis is preferable as a way of ESRD management, perception that the elderly or those with concurrent non-renal pathologies do not well after transplantation, perception that the elderly should not compete with younger dialysis patients for the limited transplant organ resource, a local dearth of cadaveric organs aggravating the limited resource competition, etc. However, data on proportion of dialysis patients on transplant waiting lists is not available for individual countries. Figure 7 shows pooled data concerning age-group distribution of European dialysis and transplantation patients, for 1988. The dialysis populations are divided into two classes, those who are *on* or *not on* a transplant waiting list. The height of each column gives the fraction of class of patient in each age group. The data are from the Combined Report on Regular Dialysis and Transplantation in Europe, XIX, for 1988. All told, only 25% of over 100,000 dialysis patients were on waiting lists. The data show that, for those who are not on the waiting list, 20% were under 45 years of age and 80% above that age – one third in the 10 year span from 55–64. One of only three reasons were cited to account for the vast majority (92%) of these – 40% were deemed to be 'unsuited', 34% deemed to be 'too old', and 18% described as 'refusing'.

Though not plotted as such in Figure 7, the percentage (%) of dialysis patients who are NOT on the transplant waiting list in each age group is: <15 years – 33%, 15–34 yrs – 25%; 35–44 yrs – 26%; 45–54 yrs – 43%; 55–64 yrs – 73%; 65–74 yrs – 90%; and over 75 yrs – 100%. As a correlate of this, the percentage of all ESRD patients, for each age group, who had already been grafted was: <15 yrs – 57%, 15–34 yrs – 49%; 35–44 yrs – 39%; 45–54 yrs – 32%; 55–64 yrs – 20%; 65 –74 yrs – 5%. Although older patients wish for transplantation less often than younger dialysis patients the chance of having their wishes fulfilled is particularly low. Thus, over 80% of dialysis patients under 50 years of age wish a transplant and have a 90% chance of eventual wish fulfilment. However, over the age of 70

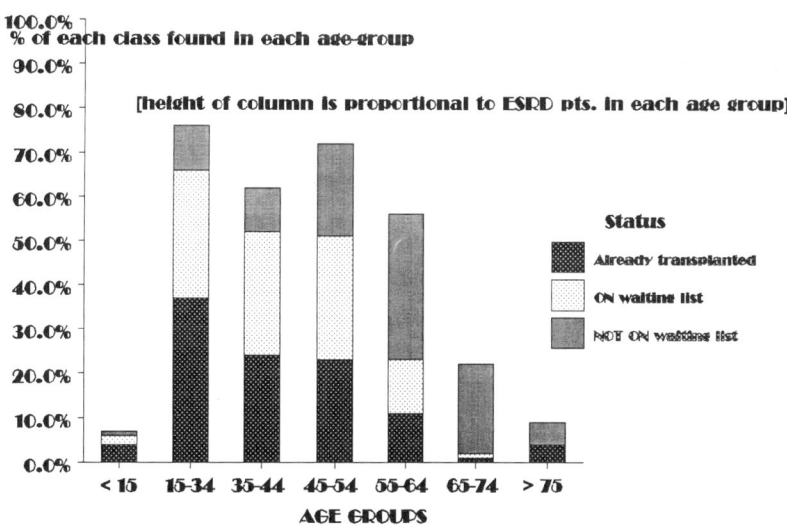

Figure 7. Three classes of ESRD patients in EDTA/ERA 1988 registry.

years, for the 20–40% who wish to be transplanted the chance of wish fulfilment is only 40% [12].

Here, also, there are many variables. They include such factors as availability of trained transplant surgeons or interested immunologists, small transplant units with somewhat inferior results, lack of physicians prepared to stimulate local cadaver organ procurement. There may also be ignorance of how good renal transplant results are in the older patient [13], etc. Also, many aspects of establishing a transplant program are poorly remunerated. Thus, 'trapped in dialysis' is only one of many factors. Nevertheless, it is probable, even in countries where many old persons (over 70) are taken on dialysis that at least 40% of all dialysis patients could be on the transplant waiting list. In areas where this is not so, it would seem ethically desirable to re-examine one's criteria.

D. *Selection of transplant recipients*

While we have written previously on the ethical dilemmas faced when choosing transplant recipients from a waiting list [14], a review of this area is in order.

Organs should be distributed to those on the transplant waiting list according to the following principles:

(*micro-allocation*)

(1) *Give organs to those most in medical need* – the 'urgency' or 'rescue' principle. This principle must be strictly defined if it is to be applied justly and must still meet minimal efficacy standards. For example, it would not be right to give an organ to an urgent case unless there was a reasonable likelihood of good outcome.

(2) *Act to optimize the medical outcome* – the 'efficacy' principle. This principle also has its ethical pitfalls. It can readily become a cloak for invalid discriminators (such as language barrier, difficulty in follow-up, anticipated lack of compliance, age, etc) masquerading as efficacy values. Even HLA typing, though of value when completely matched, is only a weak efficacy factor. HLA typing is embraced so readily as a supposedly strong efficacy factor because it places medical decision-making into a computer program which technologist can apply in the small hours of the night!

(3) *Those whose organ transplants have failed have a special claim on a second transplant* – the 'fidelity' principle. This has ceased to be a problem in renal transplants as dialysis is the better back-up to a failed graft, but it operates strongly in heart transplantation.

(4) *Allocate by random choice of recipient* – the 'lottery' principle.

(5) *Allocate using the principle of 'first come, first served'*; longest on the waiting list gets the priority. These last two principles recognize the justice inherent in chance, but deny the value of professional expertise based on medical science. It is perhaps for this latter reason that these two principles are not used much, though patients see them as just.

(6) *Allocate according to 'ability to pay'*. Historically, this has been the main factor in obtaining healthcare. It is only in the last 50 years that government has seen basic healthcare as a citizen's right (and government obligation). The factor still operates in countries which do not have mandated health insurance backed by government.

(7) *Allocate using parameters of social worth*. The experience in selection of ESRD patients for dialysis in Seattle in the 1960s, using this principle, has become a legend in medical ethics. It is now recognized as unjust.

(8) A*llocate because of the pressures of lobbying* – 'the squeaky wheel;' – this includes appeals through the media, etc. Who of us can deny the strength of this set of factors? Yet there is no question that they are the cause of much injustice.

(macro-allocation)

(9) *Recognize the needs of the program* in allocation organs to recipients. This is an undoubted factor when new transplant programs are being established. It is necessary to have success in order to consolidate funding. The principle can be ethically applied provided it is stated openly as part of public policy, so that patients are aware of it, and that it be stated as only being in operation for a limited and stated period of time.

Attempts have been made to take a number of factors into account in allocation kidneys [15], but there is no perfect system. Individual transplant units must remain aware, however, of the inherent ethical problems which they face, in this area.

E. *Ethics issues in cadaveric organ procurement*

The thrust for cadaveric organ procurement programs initially came from nephrologists interested in renal transplantation, from surgeons interested in renal transplantation, and from immuno-hematologists who became interested in the HLA region on chromosome 6. The latter group, later, also became interested in-HLA based organ allocation and distribution organizations (for examples, Paris- Scandia- Euro- and UK-transplant, SEOP, UNOS and LA-transplant).

All Western countries now accept the criteria for the determination of death from cerebral causes and also generally approve of cadaveric organ procurement. This being so, why does the transplant rate vary so widely? (see Figure 2) Whose responsibility is it to obtain these organs?

It is simple fact that shortage of kidneys for transplantation is the greatest barrier to optimized effective management of ESRD. When organ procurement rate is low and/or acceptance to dialysis is high, patients accumulate in dialysis programs. As they accumulate, there is likely to be a greater tendency to consider the older patients as 'unsuited' or 'too old', thus removing them from the competition with younger patients for the limited resource – cadaver kidneys. Although it has not been unequivocally shown that transplantation leads to greater longevity in ESRD, there is little disagreement that a) the quality of life is better after successful transplantation and that b) most patients prefer that option. It is therefore one of the most important obligations for nephrologists, in our opinion, that the transplant option be facilitated to the greatest possible extent. Indeed, one might claim that all nephrologists have an obligation actively to support cadaveric organ procurement even if their individual interests in ESRD may be in other directions. It is a duty owed to the ESRD patients whom they seek to serve. 'No man is an island' states the poet Donne, '... ask not for whom the bell tolls, it tolls for thee!'

F. *The role of the media in shaping public opinion*

Dialysis and transplantation are both programs which have elicited strong interest from both the media and from the public at large. The restoration of near death to life, and the quality and duration of life has fired the public imagination. It is because of this that governments have agreed to fund these programs.

One has only to consider the following aspects of the transplant field to realize what a crucial role is played by an informed public:

(1) Family members are expected to be able to grasp the concept of 'brain-death' in bodies which are pink, warm to the touch, have beating hearts, sustained blood pressure, and are forming urine – showing full bodily functions except consciousness and spontaneous breathing. Can such persons really be dead? How does one know that they are not in deep coma and that their breathing will come back? How much must be taken on trust!

(2) Further, these families are asked to *trust* healthcare professionals, at critical moments of life and death, when all are strangers to one another. They must trust that everything which is being told them about the irreversible nature of 'brain-death' is absolutely true, without exception.

(3) Then, these relatives are asked to consider the organ needs of strangers at moments when they are trying to cope with the frustration, the agony, and awful adjustments of unexpected and sudden death.

(4) Lastly, patients in the waiting pool of transplant recipients are asked to *trust* that their interests are being safeguarded by an equitable system of organ distribution.

Healthcare professionals become convinced about the facts of transplantation by reports in the medical and nursing literature, and by presentations at professional meetings, etc. However, the public become convinced that they can place their trust in the system only if they sense that the process has been openly reported in the press and to the media, examined by their reporters and has withstood their scrutiny.

Not all areas of medical practice need public scrutiny of this type. But both the dialysis field (because of the vast public expenditure) and transplantation (because of its unique ethical dilemmas) are two such areas. It is for this reason that nephrologists and transplant physicians need to be open with the media and be prepared to discuss plans and strategies. Our ultimate authority, let it be stressed, is not the professional association or hospital administration, but that section of the public who suffer from end-stage renal disease – they are the group who constitute our real authority to act.

Table 1. Incidence and prevalence of ESRD in various countries in 1988 (and two estimates of the chances of getting a renal transplant)

Country	Popn millns	Incidence ESRD /year /million	Transplant rate /year /million	%Chance Tx (d) as% of (c)	%Chance Tx(*) (d) as% of. 33(g)	Prevalence of dialysis /million	Prevalence of transplant /million	Prevalence of ESRD /million
(a)	(b)	(c)	(d)	(e)	(f)	(g)	(h)	(i)
USA	245	144	36	25%	26%	448	150	598
Canada	25	74.4	35	47%	52%	200	200	400
Japan	123	134	6	4%	2%	721	57	778
Austria	7.6	95.7	43	44%	52%	250	160	410
Belgium	9.8	85.2	41	48%	42%	292	158	350
F.R.G.	60.8	77	29	38%	25%	344	96	440
France	55.6	56.3	33	59%	36%	277	83	360
U.K.	56.9	55.1	31	56%	69%	136	148	284
Italy	57.4	54.7	8	15%	9%	269	61	330
Sweden	8.4	64	42	65%	75%	167	226	393
Ireland	3.6	33.8	22	65%	75%	88	138	226

(*) assumes that the % of dialysis patients awaiting Tx is 33% of all on dialysis.
(SOURCES: U.S. Renal Data System, Annual Data Report, 1990; Japanese National Dialysis Registry, 1988; Combined Report on Regular Dialysis and Transplant, Europe, XIX, 1988; Canadian Organ Replacement Registry, 1988)

References

1. Brunner FP, Brynger H, Ehrich JHH *et al.* Combined report on regular dialysis and transplantation in Europe, XIX. Nephrol Dial Transplant 1988; **4 (suppl. 4):** 5–29.
2. U.S. Renal Data System. Annual Data Report 1990.
3. Japanese National Dialysis Registry 1988.
4. Canadian Organ Replacement Registry 1988.
5. Demography of Dialysis and Transplantation in Europe in 1985 and 1986. Trends over the Previous Decade. Nephrol Dial Transplant 1988; 3: 714–27.
6. Wing AJ. Can we meet the real need for dialysis and transplantation. Brit Med J 1990; 301: 885–6.
7. Challah S, Wing AJ, Bauer R *et al.* Negative selection of patients for dialysis and transplantation in the United Kingdom. Brit Med J 1984; 288:1119–229.
8. Kjellstrand CM, Simmons RL, Goetz FC *et al.* Renal transplantation in patients with insulin dependent diabetes. Lancet 1972 ii: 4–8.
9. Shideman JR, Buselmeier TJ, Kjellstrand CM. Hemodialysis in diabetics. Arch Intern Med 1976; 136: 1125–30.

10. Brunner FP, Brynger H, Challah S *et al*. Renal replacement therapy in patients with diabetic nephropathy, 1980–85. Report of the European Dialysis and Transplant Association Registry. Nephrol Dial Transplant 1988; 3: 585–95.

11. Plough AL, Salem SR, Schwartz M *et al*. Case mix in end stage renal disease. Differences between patients in hospital based and free standing treatment facilities. New Eng J Med 1984; 310: 1432–36.

12. Kjellstrand CM, Ericsson F, Traneus A *et al*. The wish for renal transplantation. Trans Am Soc Artif Intern Organs 1989; 35: 619–21.

13. Lauffer G, Murie JA, Ting A *et al*. Renal transplantation in patients over 55 years old. Brit J Surg 1988; 75: 984–7.

14. Dossetor JB. Principles used in organ allocation. In Land W, Dossetor JB (eds): Organ replacement therapy: Ethics, justice and commerce. Springer-Verlag, Heidelberg 1991; pp. 393–8.

15. Starzl TE, Hakala TR, Tzakis A *et al*. A multifactorial system for equitable selection of cadaver kidney recipients. JAMA 1987; 257: 243–6.

4. From him that hath not

JANET RADCLIFFE RICHARDS

When the trade in transplant organs from live donors first came to public attention in Britain a year or two ago, what was most remarkable about the immediate response was its unanimity. From all points of the political compass, from widely different groups who were normally hard pressed to agree about anything, there came indignant denunciations of the whole business. The trade was an intolerable exploitation of the poor by the rich, whose greed was now invading the very bodies of those from whom there was nothing else to take. It was repugnant in every respect, and should be banned forthwith.

This indignation was not, in the first instance, directed at the worst abuses that are now known to go on. The outrage was later intensified by revelations of such horrors as kidney stealing, failure to pay the agreed price, and even abduction and murder, but these aspects of the trade did not appear until later. The trade in organs from live donors was, in Britain at least, universally denounced as unacceptable in itself, and this remarkable consensus made its subsequent prohibition by law almost a matter of form. The case for ending the trade seemed quite conclusive.

Nevertheless, I want to argue that the matter is nothing like as clear as it may seem. Of course there is something repugnant about the whole business, but it is nevertheless very far from obvious what that something is, or that it justifies the demands that the trade should be stopped. If we start not with our own feelings of repugnance, but with the situation of the exploited people on whose behalf we profess all this indignation, the matter begins to look very different, and should at least give us pause.

Consider, as an example, the situation of the young Turkish father swept to the glare of British television by the surge of outrage that followed the revelations. He had arranged to sell a kidney in order to pay for urgent hospital treatment for his little daughter. Now presumably the prospect of selling his kidney seemed, to say the very least, no less repugnant to him than it does to us, but he nevertheless judged it to be the best option available to him. This very fact shows how unspeakably bad the alternatives must have seemed. Anyone who is in favour of forbidding the trade, therefore, must recognize that the most immediate consequence of doing so seems to be taking away the best available option from people whose position is already so appalling that this is their best option. It is to make the worst off worse off still.

C. M. Kjellstrand and J. B. Dossetor (eds): Ethical Problems in Dialysis and Transplantation, 53–60.
© 1992 *Kluwer Academic Publishers. Printed in the Netherlands.*

Now this is not enough to show that the trade ought to be allowed to continue; most things we believe we ought to do can be shown to have some bad consequences. However, it does mean that anyone who wants to prohibit the trade needs to produce a very good justification for doing so. It needs to be shown either that the harm prohibition will do is outweighed by more important considerations, or, alternatively, that this harm is only apparent. Can either of these be done?

The usual justification we give for interfering with other people's actions is that we want to prevent their harming others. That, however, would be most implausible here. Far from harming anyone else, the father was benefiting his daughter, and probably saving the life of the kidney's recipient as well. (Our desire to protect the poor should presumably not lead us to conclude that the lives of the rich – people like us – do not matter at all.) If we intervene and prevent him from selling his kidney, therefore, we not only cut off what seems to him his own best option and forbid him to sell what is, if anything is, his own; in this case, at least, we also prevent the saving of two other lives. I suppose odd cases might arise in which it could be argued that prospective organ sellers were risking unreasonable harm to other people in selling their organs, but such cases are not typical. And anyway, if that were really our concern it would lead us to try to be discriminating about our prohibitions, and prevent only the sales we thought would, on balance, do more harm than good to others. Since what the sellers most obviously do is save the lives of the buyers, and frequently benefit their own dependents as well, a general prohibition would far more reliably cause harm to others than prevent it. A principle that people should be prevented from harming others, therefore, cannot possibly be used to support a general prohibition of organ selling.

Perhaps, then, the idea is to protect not other people, but the would-be vendors themselves. They are making what they regard as the best choice available, but perhaps we want to claim that they are simply misguided: that it would really be best for them to keep their kidneys and do without the money. This idea is certainly more in keeping with the tone of the popular outcry, which does, after all, express indignation on behalf of the exploited victims of the rich, and it is indeed the claim that most supporters of prohibition will produce when pressed. Nevertheless, most people will find, when they look at it, that this line of argument is just as difficult to sustain as the argument is about harming others.

In the first place, it is worth pointing out that this is not an argument that can be invoked by anyone who holds the fundamental liberal principle that even though people's freedom of action may legitimately be curtailed to prevent their harming others, it may not be curtailed to prevent their harming themselves. Anyone who takes this principle to be absolute, as many do, obviously cannot justify prohibition on the grounds that organ selling is harmful to the seller. Even if is argued that some of the potential vendors are being subtly coerced, or are too ill-informed to make rational decisions, the absolute version of the principle can justify intervention only in particular cases. It cannot permit a general prohibition which curtails the freedom of all.

Now of course that point does not apply to people who are less full-bloodedly liberal (or libertarian) than this, and who are likely to regard paternalism as justifiable in some cases. Many people – perhaps most – approve of such things as laws demanding the use of seat belts or prohibiting the use of drugs. But even supporters of limited paternalism still have to confront, in this context, the problem of explaining why kidney selling is so obviously misguided, and why a benevolent paternalist would prevent it.

Of course it is a risky business (as, indeed, is altruistic kidney giving), and no doubt in many cases, at least at present, vendors may be making choices they would not make if they were better informed, and which a benevolent paternalist would therefore want to prevent. But there is not the slightest reason to think this must always be the case. There is nothing obviously irrational and mistaken about taking risks. We do not usually regard risking life and health as absurd even for people who are rich enough to have other options open to them: normally we think it entirely a matter for individual decision if people are willing to risk their lives for the joys of rock climbing or the high salaries that go with North Sea diving. It is surely far more difficult to see why the desperately poor, who may find in selling a kidney the only hope of making anything of their wretched lives or perhaps even of surviving, should be regarded as so manifestly irrational as to need saving from themselves.

Of course many of the vendors are, in some sense, acting against their own interests. Many, like the Turkish man, are taking what risks there are for the benefit of others. It is true that the father would have been greatly distressed by the death of his daughter, but most people would nevertheless count his action as one of altruism, and taken in her interests rather than his own. Even in such cases, however, it is still not clear why a paternalist should feel obliged to intervene. Is it irrational for a man to take risks with his own life to save the life of someone he loves? Should we make a general policy of intervening and insisting on unswerving attention to self interest whenever people are tempted to sacrifice themselves for the good of others? Once again, most people would say not. And anyway, it is quite clear that most of the people who oppose the trade in organs have no such view, since they are the very people who say that only pure altruism can justify organ donation. If the daughter had herself needed a transplant, and the father had offered his kidney, they would have applauded. What difference does it make that there is an extra link in the chain, and that he sacrifices his kidney for money to save her by other means?

In one way or another, therefore, most people are going to find it very difficult to justify a general prohibition of organ selling in terms of concern for the well being of the sellers. Even if they are not opposed to paternalism on principle they still have the problem of explaining why choosing to sell a kidney is necessarily misguided, and why a well-judging paternalist would ban the trade outright rather than intervening only in particular cases.

Perhaps, then, we should try an argument based on the idea of exploitation. Even if poverty does not necessarily make people irrational, it may be argued, it certainly makes them vulnerable. We have, therefore, a duty to protect them.

No doubt we have such a duty, but if protecting the poor from exploitation is our concern, banning the trade in organs is a very strange way to go about it. An exploiter is typically someone who makes use of the fact that people who are desperately poor will clutch at even the slightest opportunity to improve their situation. Someone whose only alternative is starvation will quite rationally agree to work all day for a loaf of bread, so the exploiter takes the opportunity to get the work done without paying more; someone in grinding poverty may well be prepared to sell cheaply what others would not part with at any price, and the exploiter makes the most of the situation. Now there is of course a sense in which if we intervene to prevent the contract between exploiter and exploited from taking place at all we shall indeed put an end to the exploitation; but only in the way that we should eliminate the miseries of slum dwelling by bulldozing slums, or solve the problem of ingrowing toenails by chopping off feet. In other words, we may end the evil in that particular form, but only at the cost of producing an even worse evil for the sufferers. The simple fact is that there is no short cut to ending what is really evil about exploitation. What makes people vulnerable to exploitation in contexts like these is their having too few options, which means that the only way to improve their situation is to give them more. We can do them nothing but harm by taking options away.

The only radical cure for exploitation is the elimination of poverty. Failing that (since we lack either the will or the knowledge to do it), the best we can do for the poor is not forbid the trade but subject it to stringent controls: organize a system that completely rules out all dealings with donors or organs of dubious origin and profiteering by middlemen, get the highest price for the organs that the market will bear, counsel prospective vendors fully about both medical matters and the use of money, and provide insurance and after care. Provisionally, then, it seems necessary to conclude that this is what we should be doing. We should be eliminating not the trade, but the abuses.

It is, however, most important to emphasize that this conclusion is provisional, and to make clear the form this argument has taken.

When people are arguing in favour of some particular political conclusion what they typically do is start with some (stated or implied) moral principle which they think should be accepted, and then try to show that the policy they want to defend follows from that principle. So, for instance, someone who wanted to defend a continued market in organs might claim that everyone ought to be allowed to do whatever they like with their own bodies, and therefore ought to be allowed to sell parts of them if they wanted to.

However, the argument put forward in this paper has not taken this form. Arguments of this kind have the obvious drawback that they work only for people who already accept the principles which are being depended on, and anyone who does not like the conclusion being defended can just reject the principle in terms of which the defence has been conducted. The argument presented here is of a quite different kind, and much harder to counter because it takes as its starting point much less contentious claims, which nearly everyone involved in this debate is likely to accept. First, that preventing the trade in organs does cause harm, not only to potential recipients of organs, who will die or remain on dialysis if spares cannot be found, but also to the many vendors whose best option – not only in their own opinions, but by most people's standards – really does lie in the horrible transaction. And second, that whenever some policy has intrinsically bad consequences it must be presumed unjustified until shown otherwise.

This is a perfectly familiar idea. It is intrinsically bad to stick needles into a child, and if you announced an intention to do such a thing you would expect other people to try to stop you. On the other hand, you would also expect most people to let you go ahead once you explained that you were bent on nothing more sinister than vaccination, because most people would accept that the expected good *justified* the immediate harm. Most people (though of course not everyone) would regard vaccination as a full justification of any pain caused by the needle, but just about everyone would say that the pain should not be inflicted *without* justification.

In the case of organ selling, however, finding a justification for prohibition seems to be a much more difficult business. The policy of banning organ sales has several consequences that nearly everyone would accept as intrinsically bad: it limits the autonomy of adults, takes away the best option open to the wretchedly poor, and allows potential recipients of organs to die. But so far no justification seems to be available for allowing these evils to happen. And by this I do not mean that no one has produced a justification that would satisfy me, or would convert (say) libertarian opponents of prohibition. I mean that so far it has seemed impossible to find a coherent justification of prohibition in terms of *anyone's* principles. The problem is not, yet, of deciding whether the principles in terms of which supporters of prohibition defend their position are ones we ought to accept. It is a much deeper problem: the fact that the justifications offered do not work *even in their own terms*. The principles invoked to do the justifying simply do not do the work required of them.[1]

What the argument of this paper does, therefore, is put the onus of proof on anyone who is in favour of prohibiting rather than regulating the trade in spare parts from live donors. It takes the form of a challenge: show that what you are advocating can be given a coherent justification in spite of the considerable harm it undoubtedly causes both to potential vendors and to potential recipients, or recognize that you are willing to inflict this harm without being able to give any justification for it, and withdraw your objections to the trade.

For what it is worth, I rather hope this challenge can be met, since I find the whole business as intuitively repulsive as does everyone else. Nevertheless, once a properly critical attitude is taken to attempted justifications it is extraordinarily difficult to find any that will fare at all better than the ones already discussed.

For instance it is often claimed – as if it were self evident – that the donation of an organ should be altruistic, and that it is inherently wrong for it to be a commercial transaction. That of course still does not explain what is wrong with kidney selling when money is wanted for altruistic purposes, and raises again the question of why direct altruism should be acceptable but indirect not. But quite apart from that there is the problem of why it so unacceptable to have anything other than altruism as the motive. It may be *best* if a kidney is offered out of love by a relative, but that does not in the least suggest that what is less than best must be wrong. It is best if elderly people are cared for at home by loving relatives, but we are not usually tempted to infer from this that people who have no relatives, or who are not loved by them, should go without care rather than have it paid for. Some services to other people are performed for love, but many (including virtually all medical services) are paid for, and no one sees any harm in that. If there is a fundamental difference between services and spare parts, what is it?

A rather more promising line may be seem to be the idea that if some practice is allowed at all, people who do not really want to do whatever it is may be coerced or bullied into it. (This is one of the commonest lines of objection to voluntary euthanasia.) That, however, is true of any kind of freedom, and forbidding something altogether on the grounds that it opens possibilities for coercion is extremely difficult to justify, because it involves placing a *certain* limitation on the freedom of *everyone* in order to prevent the *possibility* of limitation on the freedom of *some*. If our concern is really to protect people who might be pressed into selling their kidneys against their will, our first impulse should be to institute a careful screening system, and refuse organs from anyone about whose motivation there was doubt. We should resort to an outright ban only after much agonizing, and after careful investigation had shown that allowing kidney trading caused more harm to people who were coerced into it than outright prohibition would cause to people who were prevented from doing what they willingly chose. We certainly have no such evidence yet.

And, moreover, even if we had, an argument of this kind could still not be used (as it frequently is) by people who are happy to condone kidney donation by relatives, since within families, surely, lies the greatest scope of all for moral bullying and other assorted pressures. If the willing and the subtly coerced can be distinguished in this context, so they can in others.

Obviously it is impossible to anticipate all the arguments that might at some time be attempted by opponents of the trade; perhaps the challenge may some time be met. My claim is not that it cannot be, but only that it has not been done so far, and that until it is done legislation forbidding organ selling is not justified. It does demonstrable harm to the worst off – the destitute and the dying – and no one has yet produced a coherent justification for allowing this to happen.

In the meantime, while opponents of prohibition continue the search for justifications, there is one general point that needs to be kept in mind. It concerns the relationship between the real reasons people have for wanting something and the rationalizations they think up afterwards.

The fact that people often have their own private motives for wanting to implement some policy does not, of course, automatically vitiate any justifications they may offer in support of it: we may often have selfish motives for wanting something that is perfectly justifiable for other reasons (as when academics and doctors protest against closure of universities and hospitals). On the other hand, it does need to be remembered that people who are firmly convinced of something are often quite extraordinarily uncritical of any argument that appears to support it.

Now one thing that is quite clear about this organ-selling issue is that the impulse to ban the practice outright was immediate and strongly felt, and not at all the result of complicated deliberations. The business was from the outset described as repugnant, and when we call things repugnant what we mean is that they produce in us feelings of disgust and revulsion. Strong feelings, however, are not in themselves reliable guides to either rationality or rectitude. Sometimes they stem from good moral impulses; but on the other hand strong feelings rooted in prejudice and superstition, and often superficially rationalized in moral terms, have been responsible for half the evils of history. We have very strong feelings about organ selling, but we are not entitled to presume that this intensity of feeling is any certificate of moral pedigree.

I do not doubt for a moment that many of our feelings of outrage in this particular context are indeed connected with the plight of the poor. On the other hand, one thing that the arguments of this paper demonstrate is that our feelings of repugnance certainly do not arise from the sources we claim, because if they did our feelings would take quite different forms.

We are inclined to say, for instance, that we find the trade in organs repugnant because of the harm it does to the vendors. But if that were really our concern we should find the idea of making their situation worse by stopping the trade more repugnant still. Since it is worse for the Turkish father to be forced to keep his kidney and watch his daughter die than sell it and save her, we should find the first situation more repulsive than the second. If we do not, it is clear that it is the sale of the kidney in itself, rather than the wretchedness of the man who is proposing to sell it, that arouses our deepest feelings.

We are also inclined to say that what we find most repugnant about the trade is the abuse and exploitation. But in that case if the trade were regulated and the donors properly paid our feelings of revulsion should go, and they show no sign of going. In fact most people would probably be even more appalled if the trade were officially sanctioned and regulated than they are by what goes on now. Or we claim that our repugnance comes from the thought that organs should be given for any other reason than love; but if that were so we should find it no more repugnant that a father should sell his kidney to save his daughter than that he should give it to her directly, and it seems we do not.

We also say, over and over again, that what we find repugnant is the way the greedy rich can take away even the little that the poor have left to call their own. But the greedy rich, in this case, are at the point of death, and the poor are being given something they value more than their second kidney. If exploitation of the poor by the rich were really the root of our deep feelings we should feel immeasurably more revolted by the unremarkable practices of everyday world trade, by which means the poor provide the rich with nonessentials and are offered only starvation wages in return. Obviously, however, we do not. We may sigh over the familiar injustices, but they cause nothing like the deep revulsion that leads to the clamour against the organ trade. Whatever we may claim, it is manifestly is not greed and inequality that really catch our deepest feelings.

It is clear, then, that our feelings of repugnance are only loosely connected with the moral principles we invoke to explain them. And from this it follows that eliminating the causes of the feelings – whatever they may be – is by no means necessarily the same thing as eliminating something that is morally repugnant.

This is most important, because it suggests one clear advantage to ending the trade that should give us particular reason for suspicion and caution as we assess putative justifications for doing so. It seems likely that if we forbid it outright we shall, for whatever reason, ease our own feelings of disgust. Prohibition may make things worse for the Turkish family and other desperate people around the world, as well as for the relatively rich who will die for lack of kidneys, but at least these people will despair and die quietly, in ways less offensive to the affluent and healthy, and the poor will not force their misery on our attention by engaging in the strikingly repulsive business of selling parts of themselves to repair the deficiencies of the rich.

Perhaps, indeed, that may in itself suggest a sufficient reason for allowing the trade to continue. If we are forced to recognize that something we find as disgusting as organ selling provides the best option for the destitute and the only hope for the dying it may help us to keep in mind the need to pursue more radical remedies: on the one hand to increase the effort to find dead donors, and on the other to take the despair of the poor more seriously.

But quite irrespective of that rather extreme justification for continuing the trade in human spare parts, one thing does seem to be clear. We must make absolutely sure that there is a better reason than the protection of our own squeamish sensibilities before we rush into legislation whose most striking and immediate effect is to take away, from him that hath not, even that which he hath.

Note

1. For a fuller discussion of the theory underlying this point see Janet Radcliffe Richards, 'Logic in the Foundations of Politics' in Logic and Political Culture, ed. E.M. Barth, North Holland Publishing Co. 1992 [forthcoming]. For a clear analysis of the problems of justification it is necessary to distinguish between what I call *formal* failures of justification, which involve a breakdown of inference between the principle invoked to do the justifying and the policy it is supposed to justify, and failures which stem from the unacceptability of the justifying principle.

5. Commercialization: the buying or selling of kidneys

JOHN B. DOSSETOR & V. MANICKAVEL

This chapter deals with the ethics of commercialism in renal transplantation. The approach will be, first, to deal with commercial aspects of unrelated live kidney donors (ULD) before moving to commercial aspects in relation to related live donors (RDL) and cadaver (CD) kidney procurement. The first poses a dilemma which besets developing countries [1], and we will use India as an example; the second and third situations pose dilemmas which are more pertinent to the developed world.

The reason for choosing India as the paradigm country for the developing world is that it has a rich and ancient religious culture, it is the country where purchase of kidneys occurs most commonly, and it is also a country towards which the authors have familiarity and much empathy. Whereas all will probably agree that Indian ethical practices are solely a matter for Indian society to work out for itself, nothing can or should prevent those in the West from wanting to understand the problem as it presents to that culture, to work up our 'outsider' positions so that each may better understand the other, and to consider *what we share as universal practices based on shared principles*.

I. Some ethics principles are universal, crossing cultural boundaries

Tristram Engelhardt, elsewhere in this volume, has discussed the question of *universality of ethics*. He points out that it is limited in extent. Nevertheless, certain principles do seem to be held 'universally' (*one should not kill the innocent; physical or mental torture is wrong; ownership of legally obtained personal property should be respected; parents hold responsibility for their children*). Even though these principles may not be absolute and may be widely flouted, the fact remains that those ethics principles which are common to all the seven main religions and to humanist philosophies could be considered to be universally held. Such common values would not include the transcendental ones, of course; these differ vastly on the basis of divine revelation even though the shared common values derive from them.

Let us consider a fundamental principle: all are equal before the law and each has a claim on society that is proportional to need. This principle of distributive

C. M. Kjellstrand and J. B. Dossetor (eds): Ethical Problems in Dialysis and Transplantation, 61–71.
© 1992 *Kluwer Academic Publishers. Printed in the Netherlands.*

justice is widely held but is expressed differently in different countries. In the West it now carries with it an *equality of opportunity* in a) primary and secondary education (but not post-secondary), b) healthcare (and, as in Canada, equal entitlement to healthcare as well as opportunity), and c) employment regardless of gender, race of minority group. Non-western countries such as India, while espousing the same principle of distributive justice, cannot extend practices of distributive justice as far. This is a reflection of an insufficiency of national resources, slower evolution of gender equality and also, perhaps, a legacy of the Hindu caste system.

If it is granted, then, that Indian society does not differ on the fundamental principles of social and distributive justice, that still does not mean that we can necessarily expect Western interpretations of social justice to be the same in India.

On examining the other four principles of bioethics: are they also shared? *Beneficence* – surely that is a shared value, indeed the duty principle of Hindu ethics to do good would be comparable. *Non-maleficence*: not to do harm, to prevent harms, to protect from harm – Hindu moral philosophy attributes great importance of this principle and extends it further in, say, attitudes towards animals than does Western moral philosophy. Their *capacity to act on it* through government policies is so much more limited that it may seem to be callously absent. Thus, there may be no government social welfare net to catch those who lose out in the lottery of life – though many individuals belong to caring extended families, the traditional security system for old age and adversity in such cultures.

It is harder to examine for the principle of individual *autonomy*. This principle has enjoyed primacy importance for less than three centuries in Western culture – stemming from the philosophy of the Enlightenment in the 17th and 18th centuries where it emerged as one manifestation of resistance to the ethic of universal subjection to the spiritual authority of the medieval church. Autonomy has enjoyed just over a century of prominence in the ethics of healthcare in the West, and has only assumed its dominance in the last 40 years. We suspect that it is only a weak principle in societies in the developing world, such as India, though the concept of group autonomy for the extended family would be stronger. However, personal autonomy is recognised there, also, as it is a necessary co-value to acceptance that all are equal before the law and are free from bondage to other persons.

Thus, we believe that Indian society shares our basic non-sectarian ethics principles and our shared dilemmas can be examined in the light of this conclusion.

II. Different rules and practices in different cultures, even when fundamental principles are shared

We are driven to conclude that sharing of fundamental principles does not mean shared practices. Practices change as a society prospers economically. The meaning given to a principle may deepen and become endowed with new interpretations as improved economic conditions enable new social horizons. (The transportation of British felons to Australia for poaching pheasants shows how much the practices of *restitutive justice* have evolved in 200 years. Yet the principle has remained unchanged throughout the intervening time.)

One hundred years ago in the West, a claim that the state should assume a duty to provide social welfare or healthcare for anyone other than custodial care for the totally destitute would have given rise to incredulity. What has changed over this span of time is government funding capacity and the public will to develop new practices of social justice. Thus, cultures which share principles may be expected to have different practices and, *between cultures*, we cannot insist on the ethical premise that 'like cases should be judged in like manner' – the rubric for issues within a single culture.

III. The autonomy model for the developing world – implications for the West

As one of the issues in kidney commerce concerns whether or not the state should restrict personal autonomy, one has to consider to what extent the principle of autonomy is altered by social conditions. What effect does poverty have on personal autonomy? Surely abject poverty, such as is seen in urban slums in Bombay and Calcutta [1] can have no equal when it comes to coercion of individuals to do things – take risks – which their affluent fellow-citizens would not want to take? Can decisions taken under the influence of this terrifying coercion be considered autonomous? Surely not. But if one adopts the view that one loses personal autonomy under conditions of abject poverty, how can one determine the level, on the scale of rising plenty, at which personal autonomy cuts in again?

It may help to divide individuals' life-goals into basic *subsistence needs* and distinguish them from basic *wants* or desires. From this position one might make the claim than those who cannot obtain basic subsistence *needs* have grossly impaired autonomy whereas failure to realize *wants* and *desires* beyond that basic level of *need* does not so do.

This leads to a view that all except those in abject poverty should be accorded the right to express autonomous choices. As for the abject poor, already fully exploited by poverty itself, they should be deemed to need societal protection – *preferably, of course, by being lifted out of poverty. State Paternalism* grounded in social beneficence dictates that the abject poor should be protected from selling parts of their bodies to help their sad lot in life. But less deprived strata of Indian society could be attributed with the right to make autonomous choices including selling body parts such as kidneys. But this argument smacks of hypocrisy. The abject poor are in such a plight that we must protect them from doing themselves harm, yet we don't use state paternalism to relieve their poverty, instead. There must be more to state paternalism than protection of a certain underprivileged class – and there is, *vide infra*.

Following this autonomy argument, there would be no reason why fully informed uncoerced individuals in Western countries should be prohibited from kidney selling to strangers. The same degree of abject poverty is no longer found there. Thus, if there is to be prohibition on kidney selling in the West – and we believe there should be – this, too, must be based on more than a state paternalistic duty to protect vulnerable citizens by overruling their personal autonomy.

IV. A review of controls by state paternalism of self-directed dangerous practices

In Western countries there are many self-directed dangerous practices in which the state shows interest in curbing the free-rein of personal autonomy. For those practices which are not (a) freely tolerated, state interests are directed at (b) imposing legal constraints to certain self-directed dangers which are still, however, tolerated, or (c) mandating self-protection in law for many everyday normal activities, or (d) eliminating the practice by prohibition. Control of kidney selling, as an autonomous act which carries some danger, would not come into either of the first two groups. The categories are:

(a) *Toleration*: Practices such as motor racing, hang gliding, rock climbing, solo ocean sailing are not prohibited, presumably because these forms of self-directed danger have no impact on others. Also, there is no indirect corrupting effect on the practitioner or others, such as with drug addiction. To prohibit them would impose excessive limitation on personal autonomy, though insisting on insurance to pay for rescues would be acceptable for some practices (taking it into the third class, below). The state tolerates unsuccessful attempts at suicide, and allows refusal of life-sustaining medical treatment by competent persons – all in the name of personal autonomy.

(b) *Self-protection Indirectly Constrained by Legislation*: Society legislates warnings of self-danger to alcohol consumers and cigarette smokers, and prohibits participation by minors. Both practices are legal, though consumption is constrained by high taxation and by warnings. Excessive drinking in public is controlled by legislation. The state also tolerates prostitution though the practice is subject to various efforts to regulate it. Yet the hidden human exploitation of prostitutes, both in earlier childhood and when practising, is known to be horrendous. Some see parallelism between kidney selling and prostitution. Both call out for regulation; many also call for prohibition.

(c) *Directly Legislated Self-protection*: Mandated seat-belts, motor-cycle helmet legislation, requirements to cross streets only at crosswalks and the rules for driving an automobile are all examples of legislation of self- and other-protective practices. For none of these, except driving, is protection of others the main motivation. The autonomy of cyclists and pedestrians is curtailed only to the extent of not ignoring the legislated self-protection.

(d) *Prohibition*: For 'street' drugs the state uses its powers of beneficent paternalism to prohibit their use, basing this on the self-unforeseen dangers of addiction and the danger of spread of addiction to others. Most Muslim and many Hindu societies place alcohol in this category, also. In the West, kidney selling to strangers is in this category though many would doubt that the practice would be comparable to addictive drug taking in its potential for harm.

Another approach to the topic is to review the types of market exchange which our society prohibits. Freedman [2] summarises the views of Walzer [3] on *blocked exchanges*, transactions which our society forbids. These are a) sales which tend to subvert the public – sale of political office, buying electors votes, b) sales which would discredit the object sold – sale of honors and prizes, c) sales of basic welfare services and civil rights – such as buying police protection, and d) sales involving desperate situations – when sellers are too easily victimized. By these standards, many believe that kidney selling comes in the fourth category.

V. Factors used to justify restriction of autonomy as regards live donor kidney selling

In the West, the argument for overriding the personal autonomy of potential kidney sellers would go as follows: (i) the *wants* of those *seeking to sell* kidneys are less than compelling, because of various social welfare systems which ensure much more than subsistent needs to all. Also, (ii) the *wants* of *those awaiting kidneys* are less than compelling. Society is providing them with dialysis; cadaveric kidney procurement programs are well financed; organ purchase is not a life or death necessity. The net benefit to sellers and buyers of kidneys is deemed not to outweigh (iii) the perceived adverse burdens/benefit of the practice to society.

The burdens to society are dealt with in the next section.

In developing countries, such as India, in contrast, (i) the *needs of those seeking to sell* may be very much greater when there is no welfare safety net, no available healthcare insurance, fewer ways of coping with the crises of life (fewer autonomous choices), greater deprivation of the needs and wants of life. Also, (ii) the *needs of those who can afford to buy* are greater because there is little alternative (no maintenance dialysis or cadaver kidney donor programs) – it is a question of a related live donor (RLD) or an unrelated live donor (ULD), or nothing. The more urgent needs of both kidney seller and kidney buyer might be deemed now to outweigh (iii) the perceived adverse burdens/benefit balance of the practice to society. This aspect will now be examined.

VI. The ethics balance of burdens vs. benefits for society

What then are the burdens to society of kidney selling, that they can outweigh the granting of autonomy to kidney sellers in the West and might not outweigh autonomy in India?

A. *Ethical burdens for society*

(1) There is repugnance, the source of which is hard to pin down, in seeing the human body treated as if it was a commodity for trade. Even the language involved in discussing kidney selling to strangers carries this repugnance. It is as if we are revolted to think that anyone can be so in need of financial aid, or value their bodily integrity so little, as to want to exchange parts of it for cash. However, this argument ignores the fact that feelings of repugnance may give place, over time, to acceptance – viz. the change in societal attitude during the last 25 years to the use of cadaveric organs for transplantation. While the repugnance is natural, by itself it is not an argument against a practice, but a factor not to be ignored just the same. A warning to move slowly, perhaps.

(2) A fundamental aspect of ethics is respect for persons collectively as well as individually. By commodifying the body, by making it an object for trade, mutual respect for all persons will be slowly eroded. This does not occur when live kidney donation is restricted to altruistically motivated relatives (RLD). The ethics of human relationships and mutual interdependency will be replaced by the utilitarian business ethics of the market place. The dignity of the human body, holistically speaking, would certainly be diminished in a way which is difficult to define, but which, at the level of community, might cause a diminution of societal commitment to altruism and human solidarity.

(3) Many, in Western society, hold a secular view that the body is different to other 'possessions'. One's whole body and mind constitutes the integrity of a self as a person. Surgical removal of diseased parts, which have come to be deleterious to the integrity of the body, is legitimate because it improves or restores the self-integrity of the body. But voluntary selling of a part which is not diseased is an offense against this holistic concept. *Indeed, a live body is not an 'it'. Live bodies are part of selves and selves are not 'its'*. The living human body holds a value which affirms our humanity as special. We should never cheapen or degrade by allowing it to be 'thingified', though we have accepted that for cadavers.

(4) Many religious traditions see the body as different from other possessions in that it is a vehicle of one's life on stewardship from God. This belief, though unsupportable by fact, is still background for our collective ethic – shared by a majority in our society. The body may be used for relief of need in those for whom we have obligations to love and support, but not sold for gain to strangers. Organ donation, in life, is only acceptable in the context of direct

altruism. (An argument for 'indirect altruism' is developed below.)

(5) In less economically developed societies, where there are wide differences in wealth, many hold that it is grossly exploitive for wealthy recipients to purchase parts of others' bodies; their wealth, it is argued, should be taxed for the needs for fresh water and improved sewerage, etc. While this argument has social appeal, the argument that they should not use their wealth for self-preservation cannot long be sustained. However, social justice might be better expressed as follows: for every individual who buys a kidney, two others from that class or sector of society from which it was purchased should receive medical treatment for renal failure, or for some similar condition which would not otherwise be treated – we have termed this aspect 'mandated philanthropy' [4].

B. *Ethical benefits for society*

(6) Our society sees its solidarity and mutual interdependency served by a realistic re-appraisal of material objects previously attributed with transcendental value. Human bodies are in this category, so the argument goes – in denial of the arguments (1) to (5), above – and should be under the control of competent individuals.

(7) The more cogent benefit is one based on *indirect altruism*. In most contemplated transactions, money is only adding a link in the chain of altruism – I wish to do good to A, my kidney cannot do good to A, but if I sell my kidney to B the money I earned from B can now be used to purchase the good that I wish for A. Although my contract with B is not altruistic, the net effect is an act of indirect altruism towards A. Individuals would have to be prepared to defend their 'indirect' altruistic desires to the regulators of a legalized kidney selling practice, in tribunals or courts. To have to defend one's motivation to others is not an infringement of autonomy, especially when other's are involved in removing and re-implanting live donor kidneys (physicians, nurses). These others have a right to know that the motivation of the kidney seller has been justified.

In settings where there is a gross disparity of wealth between kidney recipient and its provider we believe that indirect altruism (ethically acceptable for the donor) only achieves ethical acceptability for the recipient when combine with 'mandated philanthropy' – an obligation to go further than the purchase, but to provide additional relief in the form of treatment for another renal failure patient who would otherwise die, or provide funds towards a cadaveric kidney program, or both.

C. *Conclusions to this point*

(a) In our view, there is insufficient argument that personal autonomy in the West (in regard to kidney selling) should be overridden by state paternalism for the sole reason of ensuring self-protection of individuals.

(b) However, the adverse burden to benefit ratio for Western societies as a whole provides adequate reason for prohibiting commondification of the living body.

(c) Therefore, commerce in organs should be prohibited in all countries with a well developed social security net.

(d) Exceptions might be made in developing countries – they would not be compelling in more affluent countries – to accept donors' desires to enact 'indirect altruism' involving organ commerce. If so, such desires would need to be put forward and each case judged on its own merits by a panel of social peers. Before accepting such a proposal, the panel would also need to consider the question of additional 'mandated philanthropy' on the part of the recipient.

(e) The benefit/burden calculus both for live donor and uremic recipient, and for society as a whole, will differ in different cultures and decisions must be culture-specific.

(f) Individuals should not be permitted to move from one cultural region to another in order to make use of more favourable mores, elsewhere.

VII. Where does this leave countries like India?

There are two manifestations of ULD kidney commerce which may be termed: a) rampant commercialism, and b) 'rewarded gifting'. The difference between these two is in the entrepreneurial process. For the former, unregulated market forces prevail and gross injustice is meted out to the donor. In 'rewarded gifting' the transplanting institution, itself, is the agency which regulates ULD selection, and makes all the arrangements on a non-profit basis, and also is responsible for effective follow-up care of ULDs. It is assumed that this method leads to selection of 'more suitable' donors and a higher proportion of the recipient's payment reaches the ULD. We claim that this is still not acceptable on ethical grounds. For ethical acceptability, we believe that potential kidney sellers must justify their desire on the grounds of 'indirect altruism' and potential buyers must be considered for the additional social obligation of 'mandated philanthropy' – the decision being taken by a panel of society representatives.

Everyone condemns rampant commercialism. Many Indian physicians see a place for 'rewarded gifting'. Most of them argue that this is acceptable only if, in addition to follow-up care for the UL donor, there is (a) agreement that cadaveric kidney transplantation is the ultimate solution, (b) a solid commitment has been made to establish suitable facilities for handling brain-dead bodies, back-up dialysis, etc. and (c) commitment to mount and participate in publicity campaigns to encourage the use of cadaveric organs. Organ transplantation is not listed on the long list of Indian Government healthcare priorities; all this activity is in the private medical arena – as, of course, is the major part of advanced medical therapy in such countries. We advocate that the justifying arguments are taken further.

VIII. Where does this leave cultures such as the West?

The only good argument to support the practice of RLD in Western countries is direct altruism. Reports that organ recipients give special compensations or benefits to RLD donors have surfaced from time to time, but it has not been seriously claimed that these are enough to suppose that kidney donations have been thereby coerced. Indeed, the absence of coercion in RLD situation make it difficult to see why recipients should not make special recognition of their relative's gift by some sort of gift in return, if they wish. The gift in return only destroys underlying direct altruism if it is of such magnitude or nature as to be coercive.

The situation is different when considering commercial aspects of cadaveric (CD) tissue and organ procurement. Commerce in organs from dead bodies benefits only the family of the deceased. The case for 'indirect altruism' cannot be made for the dead family member, in this situation. For the family to attempt to base a claim for 'indirect altruism' – education of an orphaned child, say – on the commercial value of their dead family member's organs would be ethically flawed, in our view.

Some argue that there is a moral duty to give transplantable organs from one's dead body for the benefit of society [5]; others that legislation should enable the state to claim dead bodies if their organs can be used for others, with 'opting out' provisions for those who object [6]. The pros and cons of both contracting in and contracting out systems have been carefully delineated by Somerville [7].

Another idea is that those who register, while living, as would-be or eventual cadaveric donors should have priority in receiving organs for themselves should the need arise – also termed the Singapore model [8]. Another approach uses the concept of the 'future's market' by which financial benefit is enjoyed by the future donor of cadaveric organs, prior to death, or by his beneficiaries after death [9, 10]. The principles behind these proposals is that of a commercial contract, with profit being enjoyed by the contactor without emotional or physical risk or sacrifice.

The current situation for North American proposals is summarized in Table 1.

Underlying these proposals are several *contrasting* social perceptions or beliefs. These are that:

(a) Altruistic CD giving should be greatly encouraged and should eventually be seen as a moral duty.
(b) Intensive public education should lead to acceptance of legislation that would permit all transplantable organs to be taken at death, unless there had been prior disavowal by the deceased.
(c) Financial inducements to healthcare professionals should significantly increase CD kidney supply.
(d) Organ transplant entitlement should be extended preferentially to those who had volunteered earlier to become an eventual CD donor. But some go further in feeling that:
(e) the shortfall in CD kidneys will never be abolished without a system of fiscal

reward of, say, $1000 to donor families – though this could also depend on prior commitment by the now deceased person [11].

Table 1. Cadaver organs

---

a. Facilitated *'GIVING'*

    i. actions by health care professionals
        (1) required request, or consideration
        (2) special fees for aspects of donor procurement
        (3) cooling of organs, prior to family authorization, in order to preserve the option for altruism
        (4) duty to follow up 'donor' families
    ii. specific initiatives to increase 'giving' by individuals or their families
        (1) special recognition of donor families ('plant a tree' program)
        (2) financial consideration (compensation for expenses, only)
    iii. general initiatives for increased public 'giving'
        (1) large scale public education programs
        (2) donor cards, e.g. issuance of driving licence dependent on answering: 'Yes', 'No', or 'Do not wish to Answer' – to a direct organ donation compliance question. Donor cards are legally binding [5].
        (3) giving one's organs after death is a moral duty [5].
        (4) advance enrolment as donor gets priority for later organ needs
        (5) a 'futures' market' in organs [10].

b. Legislated *'TAKING'*

    i. Legislation which enables organs to be taken unless deceased has previously 'opted out'
        (1) 'strong' – prior statement by deceased is the only exclusion [6, 7, 8]; this would also permit cooling of organs in those who die unexpectedly and from non-cerebral causes
        (2) 'weak' – also ask for family affirmation, after death Experience in Belgium and Austria very positive [6b]

c. Possible circumstances for *'BUYING'*

    i. *special benefits* for families which authorise organ removal (non-transferable into money)
        (1) funeral grants, educational grants, etc.
    ii. *direct payment*, as money
        (1) token amounts, such as $1,000 [11]
        (2) some calculation of 'fair market value'

Ethically, the water is muddied. Contracting out systems and systems which link entitlement to enrolment in 'future CD donor' registries or futures markets favour the 'with it' population who are educated and informed. They unfairly disenfranchise less educated and less prudent citizens. For the latter a modest financial reward is deemed to be a more powerful incentive. We, in the West, should do everything to encourage the motive of direct altruism and pursue every route except that of commercialization. But we should not allow kidney selling as a manifestation of 'indirect altruism'. For less affluent areas, however, we believe it is legitimate to explore further the notion of regulated 'indirect altruism' and 'mandated philanthropy'.

In the final analysis, as in other ethics analyses, one pursues reason as completely and as far as is possible, but finally uses a resonating system of reason informed by emotion [12] – the emotion of what satisfies one's mind as feeling right. It is that emotional conviction which ultimately should determine where one makes one stand.

References

1.   Dominique Lapierre. The City of Love.
2.   Freedman B. The ethical continuity of transplantation. Transpl Proc 1985; 17: 17–23.
3.   Walzer M. Spheres of justice. New York: Basic Books 1983.
4.   Dossetor, JB, Manickavel V. Ethics in organ procurement, a contrast of two cultures. Transplant Proc 1991; 23 In press.
5.   Peters DA. A unified approach to organ donor recruitment, organ procurement and distribution. J Law and Health 3(2) 1989; 157–87.
6.(a) Hoffmaster B. Freedom to choose and freedom to lose: the procurement of cadaver organs for transplantation. Transpl Proc 17 1985: 24–30.
6.(b) Mickielsen P. In Land W, Dossetor JB (eds): Ethics, Justice and Commerce in Organ Replacement Therapy Springer-Verlag 1991; p. 191.
7.   Somerville MA. 'Procurement' vs. 'donation' – access to tissues and organs for transplantation: should 'contracting out' legislation be adopted? Transpl Proc 1985; 17: 53–68.
8.   Iyer. Kidneys for transplant – Opting out law in Singapore. Forensic Science International 1989; 35: 131.
9.   Brams M, 1977: Transplantable human organs should their sale be authorized by state statutes? Am J L & Med 1977; 183: 3.
10. Cohen LR. Increasing the supply of transplant organs: the virtues of a futures market. George Washington Law Review 1989; 58: 1,1–51.
11. Peters DA. An amended unified approach to organ donor recruitment, organ procurement, and distribution. UNOS, January Paper for discussion; 1991.
12. Callahan S. The role of emotion in ethical decisionmaking. Hastings Center Report June/July 1988; 18:9–14.

6. 'For-profit' and 'not-for-profit' dialysis: cost cutting and solutions in the USA

ALAN R. HULL

I. Introduction

Although the term profit making in medicine carries negative connotations for many people, there is little doubt that in dialysis the co-operation between industry, always willing to make a profit, entrepreneurial physicians, and recently institutions driven to find monetary support, have lead to more patients being accepted and treated in the United States than anywhere in the world. In 1989 almost 200 patients/million were accepted for dialysis in the USA, the runner up Japan accepted around 150 and there is no European country as yet who has broken the 100 pt/million barrier for the treatment of End Stage Renal Failure (ESRD).

The development of dialysis in the United States will be discussed in this chapter; the interaction between 'for- profit' and for 'not-for-profit dialysis'; the dangers of governmental cost cutting which has resulted in great efficiency, but may now pose a great moral problem for American nephrologists by forcing 'cheap dialysis'; and possible solutions to this dilemma will be suggested.

In order to consider the 'for-profit' and 'not-for-profit' implications in the development of the End Stage Renal Disease (ESRD) program, it is necessary to go back into history to events as they evolved in the late 60s and the early 70s of this 20th century. Fortunately, Richard Rettig has recently pulled together the historic events that produced the foundation for what is now the ESRD program [1]. As Dr. Rettig points out very early in his paper, 'memories are unreliable sources of details about events that occurred many years ago'. While his statement is fine it is necessary to go back to those days in order to formulate the base of the 'for-profit' portion of the program.

As a recipient of one of the 14 hemodialysis contracts awarded in 1966 by the Public Health Service (PHS), Dallas, like each of the other centers, evolved to be different and developed an approach that fitted the local needs. The grants were funded on a decreasing basis for 5 years which was one of the keys to the program's success.

The program in Dallas began to accept patients in 1968 and by 1970 it had become evident that while it was effective in serving Dallas and North Central Texas, it was ineffective in caring for the indigent patients at Parkland, our Charity Hospital.

C. M. Kjellstrand and J. B. Dossetor (eds): Ethical Problems in Dialysis and Transplantation, 73–90.
© 1992 *Kluwer Academic Publishers. Printed in the Netherlands.*

After 2 years only 2 patients were trained out of the whole Parkland system. The reasons for this were probably two-fold. First, there were not many 'Boeing engineers' to choose from the city/county hospital population. Secondly, while home training is expensive and difficult selection may have been too stringent in those early days.

Regardless of the reasons, it was clear that some other form or style of dialysis was needed to take care of the patients seen on regular renal rounds. At this time the so-called incenter dialysis units were opening in Minneapolis [2], and elsewhere. In mid-1970 I was approached by a private group made up of physicians backed by insurance companies and Ford Foundation money to open a 'store front', in-center 'for-profit' dialysis unit. This seemed to be the answer to the Dallas dilemma. On approaching the medical school and city/county hospital an unexpected obstacle was encountered. Despite the fact that it would cost the institutions nothing, and in fact they would receive rent and other support, the project was deemed unacceptable because the dialysis company was 'for-profit'. Neither institution could accept that there be *any* association between a 'non-for-profit' institution of higher learning and a 'for-profit' entity. It is amazing to look back and realize such a stand was held only 20 years ago. How long ago was it that such a view became obsolete?

II. The first step

Reason, however, finally prevailed and an outpatient dialysis center was allowed to be established.

Having overcome the initial problems a unit was developed in what was then essentially unexplored territory but there were questions as to what to charge. At Parkland, $325 was charged for a dialysis, but rarely collected. Insurance companies were unwilling in many cases to pay and Medicare did not pay, therefore, we tried to calculate cost and also include a profit. Today, one might say that that should not have been a problem, one should just set the price as high as possible. The aim in 1971 was to avoid setting the price too high for fear no-one would pay. Our hope was to 'break even' initially and later, as the number of patients increased, to allow for a profit and then lower the price.

Our initial effort was $215/treatment. If we had to see the patient at other times we charged that visit separately in addition to any laboratory costs. Surprisingly, we were able to break even and as the unit slowly grew and we began making a profit we gradually reduced the price to $185/treatment.

III. One step forward, two steps back

In 1972, Vance Hartke, a Senator from Indiana, attached a rider to a bill to pay for dialysis and transplant under Medicare. It was thought that the bill would never be passed by the whole Senate, but it was. There was speculation that the House of Representatives would never accept it, but they did. And, finally, it was felt that President Nixon would not sign it, but he did.

We were now faced with a number of new ethical dilemmas.

1. What to do about our $185/treatment price, should we reduce it further? We decided not to because the future now appeared unclear. However, there was also some concern that the Government might pay $200 and we would be frozen at $185.
2. Would the Government pay on July 1, 1973? Could we really accept all patients under Medicare? It seemed to be the impossible dream especially after all the fighting with the insurance companies.
3. Should we accept the Government money? There was however, concern expressed that perhaps we should not accept the Government largess and if we did, we might be sorry.
4. What should be done about patients who had no money until Medicare started to pay in a few months, but needed to go on dialysis now? It seemed unconscionable to allow such patients to die because of a short term monetary loss. It was decided that such patients should be accepted [3]. In February, 1973 we accepted our first non paying patient supported by the realization that we would begin to get paid in less than 5 months.

In May the government announced a price of $150 for the dialysis treatment and the physician's payment. In retrospect, an amazingly accurate choice for that time.

A. *The first ethical consideration*

With the Government paying for treatment there was now a choice heretofore unavailable to most of us. Since patients were now being covered by Medicare, should one revert to 'not-for-profit' status? This was an open choice; a doctor's contract allowed it and a nephrologist in 1973 really controlled the referral of the few patients there were. For many nephrologists faced with the prospect of opening a unit, the type of unit was a serious consideration. Since most came out of medical school settings or were closely associated, it is not surprising that many at that time chose to go the 'non-for-profit' route. Rather than an ethical decision, the choice probably afforded a simple solution with a certain comfort level.

Summary

I have opened with such a narrative review because I believe it is important for readers who were not involved in these isues in the 1960s and 70s, to understand the background from which the ESRD program has emerged.

The concept of the Government becoming a major or even sole payor was never a consideration as far as I was aware during the formative years (1970–72) of outpatient dialysis.

An unmentioned fact, with some ethical considerations, was the windfall to the insurance industry which was already starting to pay for dialysis in 1972. The actuarial allowance in the premiums was, I suspect, forgotten as insurance companies stepped back behind Medicare to secondary payor status and some companies even tried to avoid that responsibility. It is important for readers to realize the almost religious-like commitment to 'not-for-profit' and the disdain held in most areas for the concept of 'for-profit'. It must be recognized that this contempt in many circles made realistic decisions about such a major ethical issue difficult for some nephrologists in certain settings.

IV. Other possible choices

As the year 1973 passed and 1974 came and went, the Medicare program finally began paying for the care of the patient. In addition, flaws in the fragmentary legislative background became evident and were changed. It needs to be recognized at this point that no-one conceived how successful the program would become both in the number of patients who could be treated and their long-term survival. In the original home training contract with the P.H.S. mentioned earlier, we were restricted from treating patients with certain diseases, e.g., diabetes mellitus and systemic lupus erythematosus. In addition, in the first few years in Dallas we only accepted patients who had the potential to be successful transplant recipients. An evaluation of these restrictions alone quickly shows the potential that was available for expansion of the program. In 1990, diabetes composed 32% of the entering patients, and people over age 65, another 35%, with some overlap of the two groups.

These facts or future growth areas were unrecognized in 1973 and 74 as the Government's major involvement emerged. Let us look at other possible approaches the Law HR1 could have taken.

There are three major tracks that might conceivably have been chosen had there been more time taken to evaluate other considerations.

1. *No government involvement.* Labor unions and other businesses were gradually dealing directly with the insurance companies to include dialysis and kidney transplantation coverage. This would have seen a much slower growth of the program, and in the 70s many patients would have died without treatment. Assuming there was full insurance coverage by the 1980s we would still have had no way of paying for the uninsured or under insured who compose perhaps 50 million of the U.S. population. At our present acceptance rate this would have allowed 8–10,000 patients per year to die without treatment due to lack of money. It should be recognized that living patients from just this population make up a disproportionately high percentage of the current program. Even if Medicare had agreed to pay for the over 65 age group we would still be confronted with

a dilemma that U.S. citizens might not have been willing to accept, i.e., a successful chronic treatment that was totally limited by lack of money. Since it was one of the major agreements allowing passage of the Hartke amendment in the first place, some intervention by states or the Federal Government might have occurred.

The result would have been a much slower growth of units and many patients dying without treatment.

2. *Limited government involvement.* There were many things poorly thought out in this time when America still believed it could pay for anything that was really worthwhile. What if Medicare had stepped in as secondary payor for those with insurance and covered only those who had no insurance or were over 65 years of age? Such a move would have been much more reasonable and would have left the ESRD program somewhat less vulnerable to many of the cutbacks that have since taken place. Why this was not done is a cogent question. I believe there were three principal reasons:

(a) This was really early in the application of the Medicare concept and it was still not clear how great the costs of an all inclusive coverage for even those over 65 years of age might be. The effect of adding to this population the disabled and ESRD was just underestimated because of too little experience. Also, cost estimates for dialysis and transplantation did not initially include other coverage for the under 65 age group, e.g., coronary artery bypasses.
(b) America despite the Vietnam War and perhaps because of President Johnson's 'Butter and Bullets' analogy, still felt it could handle these kinds of problem for the overall good of its citizens. Maybe there was a feeling that the end of the Vietnam War would free up additional monies to allow great things to be done. In this case the American optimism may have bitten off more than it was able to chew, let alone digest.
(c) In my reading I find no consideration for what was already being paid for. Rettig[1] estimates that there were 10,000 patients on dialysis in 1973. The majority of these patients were being covered by insurance payments or they could not have been dialyzed. This oversight seems to me to be a major one that has never been explained. Medicare in early writings always stated that there was no market. This is not true, there was a market but it was ignored. As a result of this oversight, Medicare was left with the whole plate and the insurance companies took their premiums which were actuarially accounted for and stole away.

If there had been more discussion, a plan which would have included private insurance with government support should have evolved, and the ESRD programs would have been more like other areas of Medicare today. One must note, however, that it would still have required Medicare coverage of the uninsured under 65 years of age and this might have been difficult to pass or envision in 1972.

3. *Government does all but with very rigid oversight.* Despite other possible ways in which Government could have become involved this is what has actually evolved. There is no going back but the rules that were developed raised some interesting ethical questions with regard to 'for-profit' and 'not-for-profit' units.

V. The concept of profit

What evolved in the ESRD program under Medicare must first be credited with what it has accomplished, before anyone points out the deficits and dilemmas.

By having the Government becoming so involved in U.S. medicine with its *'laissez-faire'* fee for service system, we have reached the following pinnacles of achievement:

1. The U.S. still has the highest acceptance rate for patients on dialysis [4] (> 170/million population in 1989).
2. Up until 1986 or 1987 we accepted more older patients on average than any other country [4, 5].
3. Even now we take more patients in the over 75 years of age group and have essentially no competition in the over 85 group [4, 5].
4. Until recently 1988 we have equalled Scandinavia in having the highest number of kidney transplants/million population and are still ahead of many other countries [7].

These accomplishments cannot be overlooked in the U.S. approach to ESRD. How our costs compare to other countries is not as clear since we keep track of them as a single program and other countries merely incorporate them in their overall health care costs, where it is a relatively small total item. This may seem strange to American readers, but in the U.S. itself, private insurance has no information on their total outlay for ESRD. However, I would speculate that the cost/patient in the US is much less than in the Federal Republic of Germany [7] or Japan [8], where facility payments are 2–3 times that of the US.

If the U.S. reimbursement is actually less, what role has the profit motive played in this alleged cost savings. At the start of the program, physicians wanting to become involved could go either way. If one were to go back to 1973 and a physician was completing his/her fellowship the choices were as follows:

1. *Initiate a program on one's own.* The major problem to this approach was that one had to have financial backing. If there was no ready support from individuals, either entrepreneurs or individuals concerned for patient welfare, nor support from Kidney Foundations or other entities, then the nephrologist had to turn to normal financial sources. This meant signing on a note at a bank, if a willing institution could be found. This lack of ready financing in the early to

mid 70s forced many to remain with medical schools and other institutions that retained unit ownership and any profit that resulted.

2. *Join or unite with a 'for-profit' group or organization.* This really took two forms. The major one probably was to become part of a physician group that owned its own unit(s). Early on there were few of these groups, but later on this number increased as it became evident that unit ownership was a viable option. Another choice was to go with a 'for-profit' chain and develop a practice where the physician wanted to establish clinics.

3. *Stay with medical school or hospital programs.* In this arrangement one admitted patients and/or become the medical director. This choice in the early times was easier, but appears to have lead to frustration as many nephrologists who started this way apparently became disenchanted and accepted options 1 & 2 above. The reasons for the frustration were many and varied.

Table I. Comparison of number and % of center types. 1981 vs 1989

		1981	1989
For-profit (all types)		416 (36%)	1018 (53%)
Non-for-profit		569 (50%)	752 (39%)
Other		158 (14%)	161 (8%)
	Total	1143	1931

Modified from USRDS 1990 report [9]

Table II. Location of patient by %. 1980 vs 1988

	1980	1988
Free standing for-profit	39	51
Free standing not-for-profit	12	12
Hospital facility	5	6
Hospital centers	27	20
Dialysis and transplant centers	17	11
	100	100

Modified from figure 14, September 15, 1990 USRDS gold notes [10]

As time passed more and more units became 'for-profit' as shown in Table I [9], and more patients were dialyzed in such units, see Table II [10]. The reason always given was that there was so much money to be made. However, there does not appear to be any good supporting data for this statement, only rumours and anecdotes. Regardless of how much money was made, and regardless of other reasons, the American system moved steadily toward 'for-profit' free standing units. Ownership was either by individuals or organizations. The organizations were mainly 'for-profit' corporations and in the most successful ones there was a profit share arrangement with certain physicians. There were also hospitals that set up such free-standing units under their 'for-profit' wing. If we look at the effect of the trend and utilize the Government figures for the early 80s we find the following results:[11]

	Median	Range
Cost For Independent Units	$108	80–214
Cost In Hospital Based	$135	86–227
Cost For Home Dialysis	$ 87	63–156

If one uses these numbers recognizing the inherent problems of obtaining such actual figures it appears evident that independent (for-profit) units had a much lower cost than hospitals (not-for-profit). The reason is always given that more attention is paid to cost in a 'for-profit' unit. This appears to be especially true when the 'not-for-profit' unit is part of a large hospital and costs are allocated for non dialysis functions. However, this provides no rationale for the government keeping the price high to hospital units.

VI. The cost reports

The Achilles Heel of the ESRD program is and has been the cost reports [11]. In order to try to determine what should be paid, the Federal Government since the middle to late 70s has depended on what is called 'the ESRD Facility Cost Report'. This is submitted each year by all facilities and is utilized from time to time to estimate the cost of dialysis. Unfortunately for dialysis units this document is based on Medicare rules and not reality. For example no allowance is made for bad debt, and up until recently there was a $32,000 limit on what could be paid to a medical director. These factors and others, allow anyone who surveys the cost report to form a totally false idea of what incenter dialysis really costs.

The Government looks at the cost report and determines that there is a profit. This concept is confirmed because units continue to open up. What HCFA and Congress have failed to recognize is that there are other reasons to open a unit even when one loses money. Let me list just two:

1. Hospitals will supplement a dialysis unit for a number of reasons:
    (a) They are willing to pay for the prestige of having a unit.
    (b) They recognize the patient need and are willing to supplement the loss from other profit centers, e.g. admission of ESRD patients for access procedures.
    (c) Some hospitals do not do careful cost accounting and as yet are not really aware that they are losing money.
2. Nephrologists may well supplement their unit from the physician's payment component. Why would a physician do this? Well the answer is really rather simple. Without the ability to do dialysis, and particularly to care for such patients when admitted to hospital, there is no specialty of nephrology to

support the number of nephrologists that have been trained. Expressed another way, if we could transplant all the ESRD patients, there is not enough routine non dialysis renal disease to keep a majority nephrologists practising nephrology. Therefore, in order to maintain a viable specialty nephrologists must have a unit and patients to take care of, and therefore they will supplement the unit to keep it open. There are at least two ways they do this:

(a) They manipulate their hospital to keep a unit open and agree to do other jobs for the hospital.
(b) They act as medical directors and provide oversight for a low price or often for free.

These approaches allow units to remain open, but the actual cost of what is provided is never correctly calculated.

Finally, by surveying only the cost reports HCA has not realized that most hospital units and many free standing units could not survive on the 80% Medicare actually pays. These units remain open by ordering ancillary drugs and by cost shifting to the private sector during the first year, now 21 months for those patients with private insurance and then collecting the 20% coinsurance thereafter. Until the Government agencies recognize these facts, patients are going to suffer as various necessary items including length of dialysis are cut back to keep units open.

VII. The ethics of profit

In the early days of the program most people involved in dialysis were rather inefficient.

1. Very few if any units reused dialyzers.
2. The personnel hired to cover shifts were mostly nurses.
3. The staff to patient ration was 2:1 or 3:1 at the extreme.

As the reimbursement decreased from $138 to $127 and lower and no allowance was made for inflation, some of these things had to be modified in order for units to survive. Many of these changes occurred first in the free standing and/or 'for-profit' units. Today, units have probably attained maximal efficiency and are now being forced to cut things that are beyond efficiency, raising an ethical concern.

A. *The early stage*

In the period 1973–1979, the decision to be involved in a 'for-profit' or 'not-for-profit' practice carried no true ethical consideration, although many people thought it did. It was frequently possible in Dallas to get more for the patient and staff in a 'for-profit' setting than in a 'not-for-profit' scene, as 'for-profit' administrators knew what the bottom line was and what the profit really was. In the hospital

82

setting, while they received a much higher payment, there was often little money available for extras. Physicians were told at payments of $250/dialysis that the hospital was losing money. As stated previously hospitals tends to load in all kinds of unrelated overhead to dialysis because that was how Medicare paid.

Summary

In the early years of the ESRD program the choice of 'for-profit' vs 'not-for-profit' really did not raise a true ethical dilemma to the forceful physician who demanded the best for his/her patients. Note the addition of this last caveat because an indecisive physician who did not 'fight for the best' was overrun in either system.

B. *The middle period*

In the period 1980–84, as payment was reduced and no allowance was made for inflation, physicians recognized that there was now pressure to cut back on patient care. The easy approach here was to dialyze in a 'not-for-profit' mode. The reason for this is evident if one looks at the legendary 'strong' nephrologist. Before the hospital rate was reduced in 1983 there was much more leeway in the hospital based setting to deliver additional care. During 1980–82 freestanding units felt the pressure of inflation since they were receiving only $138 and therefore became used to innovating. In 1983–85 'for-profit' units also had a payment reduction ($138 to $127 on average) but this reduction was not as severe as the average decrease for hospitals ($159 to $131). Here a true ethical dilemma evolved: How could you maintain good patient care while still making a profit in which you shared? The rationale had to be how well are the patients doing and what would happen if care consumed all the profit. The second part of this was often not analyzed. If all the profit was used for patient care the unit would have to close. There was no hospital backing for most freestanding 'for-profit' units to shift costs to. Faced with the tension of closing vs maintaining patient well-being, most nephrologists did what I believe was the best job possible. Held *et al.* [12] and Wolfe *et al.* [13] have not been able to show any difference in patient survival or in other measures. After 1983 the 'for-profit' units began to take up the developing slack as growth continued and more and more units of that type were opened. The reason was often said to be greed and the desire to make money, but I do not accept that thesis. Hospitals had the same ability plus $4 more yet they began to back away, see Tables I & II.

The means whereby 'for-profits' and their nephrologists accomplished this was by slowly expanding and experimenting with the dialysis process. I still remember our apprehension with every change, reuse, different staff ratios, and shortened time. In every case this appeared to be successful, at least when results were compared between sites in the United States. Finally, not that it means anything or verifies it, but hospital and 'not-for-profit' units followed the lead of the 'for-profits' as inflation and other cut backs continued.

Summary
From 1980 to 1985 many changes evolved in dialysis in order to allow an ever increasing number of patients to dialyze. It was a time in the early part when hospital units being paid more had a chance to do more and increase, but unfortunately they did not. The question however remains, should one modify patient care and still make a profit. I believe the answer is 'yes' as long as patients are aware of the situation and the physician believes the care he/she is offering is as good as is available. You will note I said available because from this time on in the ESRD program and particularly in the later period I believe it was possible to offer better care had there been more money available. The 'for-profit' physician treads a very fine line in this tension between what is adequate profit to keep units open, and what is good care, and when he/she feels that profit has gotten out of hand he or she must quit or demand changes.

C. *The current period*

This covers from 1986 to the present. In this time frame all physicians are caught in the ethical dilemma of taking care of increasing numbers of patients with inadequate reimbursement. This now effects nephrologists in the 'not-for-profit' as well as the 'for-profit' sector. Now the ethical dilemma has changed and this change must be recognized. In many hospital units, despite physician requests and demands, the units cannot be expanded to meet the 9%/year increase in the patient population. These doctors face an ethical dilemma in that their own patients have to be denied care or be referred elsewhere because of lack of space. The 'for-profits' ethical dilemma is somewhat different. Besides the profit question the freestanding 'for-profit' physician knows that his or her unit may be able to continue to expand because there is a profit and without the profit many patients will die because expansion will not occur. However, both groups of physicians should now recognize that our care of dialysis patients may well be suffering not because of profit, but because the Government does not pay enough for adequate care. This ethical problem cannot be solved by nephrologists speaking out because the Congress and HCFA always see physicians input as self-serving. Only when the patients stand up as a group and demand better patient care and the reimbursement necessary for such care will something be done.

Summary
In the current period 'for-profit' and 'not-for-profit', hospital units and freestanding units are underpaid. The 'for-profit' sector is the only one expanding to any extent. This does not justify 'for-profit' but it does again demonstrate that the profit system often allows things to be done that will not or can not be accomplished under other systems.

VIII. The systems in the rest of the world

Having reviewed the dilemma of the US system and the ethical choices, let us now turn and compare the US to elsewhere. The reader should recognize that I have not worked in most of these countries, and therefore, my comments are that of a distant observer.

A. *Japan [8]*

I am told the Japanese units are most often physician owned and payment appears to be on an incentive basis. By incentive I mean they receive more if they dialyze longer, dialyze at night or use a bigger dialyzer. Of course, I happen to favour such a program and it appears to have worked well in Japan. However, Japan has a number of insurance programs that pay for dialysis with the government as a safety net. Finally, Japan does not have our current budget problem which essentially drives the US Medicare system. At 130 yen to the dollar their reported payment approached three times that of the US.

B. *Federal Republic of Germany [6]*

Up until the reunification of Germany, the German social insurance plan paid for dialysis (both the physician and the facility component). It has always been unclear what percentage of German dialyzing nephrologists are on salary and how many are on their fee for service system. However, data available suggests overall payment approaches twice that of the US.

C. *Scandinavia*

According to Kjellstrand [6, 14] the system is totally socialistic with no fee for service and no incentives for seeing more patients. The system appears to encourage inefficiency and does not encourage physicians to see more patients or seek referrals.

D. *United Kingdom*

The system in the United Kingdom has been restricted by financial rationing. Dialyzing physicians are on salary and there tends to be a financial cap on the number of patients they can accept, hence the push toward transplant and CAPD. In my short time in England spent at major teaching hospitals, I was impressed with how well the system worked without real incentives. I was told, however, that many patients who could benefit from dialysis were not referred to the tertiary hospitals with dialysis units. Once at such hospitals, patients seemed to be accepted by the same criteria as in the US.

E. *Canada*

The Canadian system varies from province to province with physician payment tending to be fee for service with financial caps. Facility dialysis, is if I am not mistaken, all hospital associated even when it is free standing.

F. *Elsewhere*

I have no real information. The 3rd world countries do not really offer dialysis in the manner we are used to. The former communist block countries accepted few patients and it was hard to recognize any plan during my visits there.

Table III. Comparison of the Six National Registries for 1987/1988.

	Acceptance (no./mp/yr 1987)	Prevalance (no/mp/ on Dec 31, 1987)	Transplant (no/mp/yr 1987)	Gross Mortallity (%)
Canada	71	186	32	18.9
FRG	76	320	27	10.0
France	56	254	24	7.3
Japan	137	671	< 2	8.8
US	151	403	37	23.4
Australia	48	152	25	13.5

If one looks at what has resulted elsewhere in the world (Table III)[4] one can see that the US still leads in patient acceptance, and is tied in the number of patients transplanted/million population. When one moves to prevalence USA is losing ground due to a high mortality rate. The 'for-profit' motive which now is (or is becoming) the major form of dialysis, therefore, may be responsible for our increased acceptance. The ethical problem here is are we now accepting patients that would not be accepted elsewhere, and can we continue to care for them adequately long term?

The US takes more patients in the > 75 age group and we are certainly unchallenged in the over 85 year section, but this is of course a very small number. As to what role our legal system plays in physicians believing they can't say no when the Government pays, is not certain. I suspect it plays a role, but I doubt it is a major factor.

IX. Other ethical dilemmas in the ESRD program

Congressman Forney (Pete) Stark, along with Arnold Relman, the former Editor of the New England Journal of Medicine, have raised the question of the ethics of nephrologists referring to their own units, and self-referral is indeed an ethical consideration. Is it, however, any more of a dilemma than that which patients and physicians face elsewhere in medicine? The common practice is for an internist or family practitioner to admit a long-term patient to hospital who subsequently manifests with heart disease and perhaps an M.I. In such situations a cardiologist of the patient's doctor's choice is consulted and often subsequent care both in the hospital and afterwards is directed by the cardiologist. In other words the patient becomes part of the cardiologist's practice. Patients who develop or are found to have End Stage Renal Disease are handled in a similar fashion. The ownership issue in a dialysis unit differs only in frequency of treatments and is on a par with the cardiologist's office and cardiac catheterization in an outpatient unit in which he or she is an owner or shareholder.

In summary I see the referral to a physician owner very little different than other areas of medicine, and at least in dialysis the treatments are limited in number and price, which may not be true for these other areas. The question may then be asked is all medicine wrong in such approaches as Dr. Relman has suggested. That issue is more relevant but also more complex. This chapter is not the place to discuss this issue, but let me conclude on this subject by saying that it seems essential that ownership be out in the open and both the referring physician and the patient should be aware of the situation. I believe most physicians do recognize ownership and it may well influence referral, and if so, that is proper. My experience is that 99% plus of patients don't find this a problem. What patients want is good care and they usually end up putting all their trust in their original doctor who referred them. Providing the nephrologist is perceived as caring and 'appears to know what he/she is doing' most patients seem satisfied. However, it must be recognized that in medical care patients are not usually given a choice regarding referral to 'for-profit' or 'not-for-profit' entities nor salaried or fee for service physicians.

X. The basis of our ethical dilemma

Physicians always have to make the ethical decision in how often they see patients, i.e. it should be influence by the patient's needs; it should never be influenced by the needs of the physician. However, that does not appear to be the source of conflict in the ESRD program since patients' needs are quite clear: they need dialysis at least 3 times/wk.

Now the problem in ESRD has taken a different turn because we have a monopsonistic purchaser which has produced far different ethical pressures and quality results. In an article in JAMA of April 11, 1990, Michael L.Ile, J.D. [15] has reviewed how monopsony can affect and in fact disrupt a market. I think it is important for us to understand this concept as Ile applies it to health care. We are all familiar with the word monopoly which is defined in the Random House Dictionary as 'exclusive control of a commodity or service in a particular market or a control that makes possible the manipulation of price'. Most commonly we think of this as in the case of an electrical company in a city. Utilities are given a monopoly but there is a controlling board which overseen prices and service.

Monopsony is defined as the market condition that exists when there is one buyer. This definition describes rather well the role Medicare plays in the ESRD program, i.e. exclusive control of the demand for a product by being essentially a single purchaser of that product Initially this seemed to work well and restricted the price increase. However, as Ile points out, that which always happens with monopsony occurred, 'the dominant buyer restricted output and caused resource misallocations'.

Normally what happens in a monopsonistic situation is that 'suppliers who are compelled by a monopsonist to accept less than a competitive price for their goods will use their assets to produce goods that can be sold for a competitive price in another market'. This is exactly what has happened in the ESRD program since 1984.

1. Physicians cannot get out of the market because patients are their livelihood.
2. Nephrologists therefore continue to care for dialysis patients in the units but put less effort there because the price is so low. In a recent talk at the American Society of Nephrology Meeting, Sam Their [16], the Director of the Institute of Medicine, gave the following price comparisons:
   (a) Dialysis unit payment has decreased from $138 in 1974 to $125 in 1989. However, when adjusted for inflation this is less than $54 in 1974 dollars, a 61% reduction.
   (b) Physician payment from 1974 to 1983 when the Monthly Capitation Payment (MCP) system was established was unchanged at a national average of $185/month. Since then it has decreased to an average of $173/month.
   More important, when adjusted for inflation over this period this is approximately $77/month in 1974 dollars. One needs to also remember in the case of patients with Medicare only and no coinsurance, that the payments are 80% of these amounts.
3. As Ile predicted, nephrologists have moved to other markets, i.e. in hospital care is still under fee for service rules and payments have continued to increase with inflation. This appears to me to be where most nephrologists put their time and effort.
4. One additional item of interest is that cost shifting to third party insurers has been allowed in the first year for patients with group insurance. While physicians and dialysis facilities have utilized this as a means to recoup for the restricted Medicare payment, and have in most cases increased charges and collections, they have been unable or unwilling to set up a two-tie system where patients with insurance get better, or longer dialysis. Instead all patients are dialyzed the same regardless of what they are paying.

It would be my personal contention that the Federal Government's position as a monopsonist has, quoting Ile one final time, 'reduced the volume of goods (dialysis) and service (physician care) provided to society by limiting the price sellers receive'. I have been asked by Dick Rettig [16] what I would suggest to remedy the situation if I really believe this is true, which I do. Since the Federal Government is deeply in debt and will probably continue that way, it is essential to remove the ESRD program from the federal budget. This is necessary because quality and innovative programs are not possible nor are ethical considerations primary when budget reduction is foremost in Congress's mind.

The ethical solution would be to get the Federal Government, as much as possible, out of the program.

A. *Solutions*

1. On January 1, 1993 Medicare would cover all people 65 years and older who are Medicare eligible.
2. Medicare would be responsible for all patients enrolled in the program on December 31, 1992. This would include those dependent on Medicare as of that date and those who have third party insurance. Medicare would pick up the latter group when their insurance ran out.
3. All new patients would be covered as follows:
   (a) Medicare would cover those who enter over 65 or those who do not have private insurance when they later turn 65.
   (b) Private insurance would cover all who have such policies until they reach age 65 and/or their insurance stopped.
   (c) All others would be covered by state programs or Medicaid.

The problem with this proposal is apparent: solution 3C. This would put an increased burden on states and some patients in economically less well off states could actually suffer. The ethical question one has to ask is: would the end result be worse for the program than the present ratcheting down (even with the $1 increase in 1991) which allows patients to be accepted but then to get inferior care, i.e. short dialysis as the program is strangled by inflationary pressures? It seems as much an ethical dilemma in this program to recognize that rationing by price has actually been applied.

XI. The final answer to these difficult questions

I have tried in this chapter to trace the history and point out where various ethical questions have arisen. Hopefully I have shown that despite discussions there were few true ethical dilemmas in the early days. Unfortunately, significant ethical tensions now apply and nephrologists must face them and speak up. I believe we have no choice at present other than to follow the 'for-profit' system because it is the only one opening new units to care for an expanding patient population. I have expressed my view that the payment monopoly or monopsony that Medicare has must be broken. However, that leave us with two current dilemmas 1) what does a nephrologist who is merely working in a facility do now when he/she sees patients are not receiving adequate dialysis? If another unit with better care is available should they move or offer their patients that choice? Usually, these options are not available, but if they are, they must make such a hard choice. 2) What does a participating nephrologist or owner do when he/she sees that dialysis in inadequate? First, they must determine if the profit is unreasonable, or if it is what profit is required in order to keep expanding and accepting new patients. A good test of this situation is: are there other units giving better dialysis? If there are then I think one has to consider carefully what the profit is and if more money should be going to patient care. The final test of all this is: Is the physician willing to let the fact that he/she is profit-sharing be made known? It would seem that if one needs to hide what is going on, there may be a serious ethical question. However, if the referring physician, the patient and staff know that a profit is being made and that the unit is superior due to this fact, then the ethical issue may be, can that physician accept patients when no one else can?

The ESRD program is an interesting one to compare in this manner to medicine at large. If the ESRD program has been able to maintain quality while reducing the cost/patient when the rest of medicine is going in the opposite direction, then medicine has some ethical questions to answer. On the other hand, if quality has suffered in order to produce necessary marginal care then the ESRD program is the place for ethical questions. Finally, if other countries pay more and accept fewer patients but produce better quality, maybe HCFA needs to evaluate what they are getting when they reduce reimbursement.

References

1. Rettig, R A. Origins of the Medicare disease entitlement. The Social Security Amendments of 1972. In Hanna K (ed): Biomedical Politics Washington D.C., Academy Press 1991: pp. 176–208.
2. Shapiro, FL, Messner R, Smith, HT. Satellite haemodialysis. Ann Intern Med 1968; 69: 673–84.
3. Hampers Constantine. Personal communications.
4. Hull, AR, Parker TF. Introduction and summary of the proceedings from the morbidity, mortality, and prescription of dialysis sumposium. Dallas, Texas, September 15–17, 1989. Am J Kidney Dis 1990; XV (5): 375–83.
5. Brunner FP, Selwood NH. Results of renal replacement therapy in Europe 1980–87. Am J Kidney Dis 1990; XV (5) 384–96.
6. Kjellstrand C, Hylander B, Collins AC. Mortality in dialysis – On the influence of early start, patient characteristics, and transplantation and acceptance rates. Am J Kidney Dis 1990; XV (5): 483–90.
7. Brunner F. personal communications.
8. Odaka Michio, personal communications.
9. United States Renal Data System. Annual Report 1990; p. 68.
10. United States Renal Data Systems. Gold Notes, Figure 14, September 15, 1990.
11. Federal Registry

12. Held PJ, Bovbjerg RR, Pauly MV *et al*. Effect of the 1983 composite rate changes on ESRD patients, providers, and spending. Urban Institute: Washington D.C., December 21, 1987.
13. Wolfe RA. Port FK, Hawthorne MV *et al*. Comparison of survival among dialytic therapies of choice in center hemodialysis vs continuous ambulatory peritoneal dialysis at home. Am J Kidney Dis 1990; XV: 433–440, May.
14. Kjellstrand CM, personal communications.
15. Ile M. When health care payers have market power. JAMA 1990; 263 (14).
16. Rettig RA, personal communications.
17. Their S. Presentation, invited lecturer at the American Society of Nephrology, Washington, D.C., December, 1990.

7. Physicians and industry: can professional integrity be maintained?

I. Conflicts of interest

How much time should one spend with a sick and needy patient when other patients are waiting? How much should one charge for one's services when the cost then excludes the poor or uninsured from having the service? How does one balance the demands of patients or academic ambition against such other values as 'time with one's family'? Such conflicts of interest are part of every professional's life; they are ethical conflicts between one's own interests and those whom one seeks to serve or to whom one has obligations.

For the health care professional, however, a special form of ethical conflict may arise when intensively promoted interests of the pharmaceutical industry (legitimate interests, as perceived by the industry) cause ethical tension between personal desires and professional obligations, in such a way that professional standards may be compromised. Important statements have been made on these issues by the Royal College of Physicians, London [1], the American College of Pysicians [2], and by some specialist groups [3]. This type of conflict is difficult to define [4], and there is greater hazard when the physician holds a position of public trust for administering programs – at the meso- or macro-level of resource allocation – than when similar tension develops with individual patients (or at the micro-economic level). In the former situation, the greater potential for private advantage (budgets are greater, more persons are involved) is no longer balanced by the stabilising effect of the direct fiduciary relationship which exists with individual patients.

In medical research, ethics in relation to industry involves the researcher in such issues as: direct funding which evades the full rigors of the peer review system; restrictions on the publication of data; pressures to emphasize matters relating to commercial implications of data; financial reward which is not commensurate with the amount of time invested; excessive rewards in 'kind' if not in 'cash'; and, risk of inadequate disclosure of the researcher's activities to legitimate authorities. All these are additional to the usual ethical obligations towards research subjects: to be selected fairly; to maintain confidentiality; and to obtain fully informed consent. The obligations are clearly outlined in the Council Report for Scientific Affairs and the Council in Ethical and Judicial affairs of the American Medical Association [5].

C. M. Kjellstrand and J. B. Dossetor (eds): Ethical Problems in Dialysis and Transplantation, 91–100.
© 1992 *Kluwer Academic Publishers. Printed in the Netherlands.*

Whereas there is little doubt that every physician knows that conflict of interest will occur in daily practice, evidence shows that MDs are insufficiently prepared for encounters with pharmaceutical representatives (PRs) [6].

Nevertheless, everyone acknowledges that the pharmaceutical and medical device industries are essential to treatment, especially as regards dialysis and trans-plantation of renal failure patients. Enormous benefit has accrued to patients from the entrepreneurial activity of these industries based on either their own research (especially in the field of drugs) or their response to medical need (especially in the field of devices). One would expect that such business would bring profits, possibly enormous profits, when a product competes successfully in the market. It is also natural that commercial companies would wish medical collaborators and see no reason why such physicians should not be well rewarded for their collaboration.

A. *The ethics of gift-giving and receiving: establishment of social and professional contracts*

Gift-giving has a clearly recognized role in our society, indeed, in all societies. Gifts obtain their meaning from sentiments shared between donor and recipient which may be difficult to express in other ways. Such sentiments include gratitude of various sorts, expressions of social and professional solidarity and even simple friendship. Gifts are designed to give pleasure. They often express an element of self-giving beyond the limits of duty or the business contract. But, in addition to improving relations between people, gifts always generate an obligation for reciprocity of some sort. Persistently unrequited or unacknowledged giving may reflect unusual affection for a person, the giver being recompensed by inner sources of satisfaction, but this is not the sort of sentiment which underlies gift giving between industry and professionals.

In the West we recognize that gifts may serve to a) show simple gratitude, b) serve as symbolic payment for past benefits or recognition of past-indebtedness, c) forge new social relationships, and d) create new indebtedness. Gifts are often disguised. This enables both donor and recipient to be inconspicuous, except to each other. Gifts may also be ostentatious or even flamboyant, such as trips to exotic places for meetings of company consultants. Gifts may be purely functional such as the gift of equipment which is only required for a limited time and could have been loaned or rented; or disguised as extension of a salary for periods longer than required for a given project, for example.

In all these transactions the concern which must be addressed is: *at what level of gift giving does the recipient's scientific objectivity or personal or professional integrity become compromised?* Carl Kjellstrand suggests the following as a sensi-tive 'litmus test': Would you be proud to have the gift publicly acknowledged on the front page of your local newspaper? It is a good one, consistent with the ethic of public accountability for those in positions of public trust. An experience of the writer is worth mentioning. It concerned consultancy conferences for a company making dialysis equipment and fluids. Each annual symposium was sited in a tropic paradise (for self, and accompanying spouse or significant 'other') at which consultant fees were earned for medical advice in addition to all travel and accommodation expenses. How could one seriously maintain that this was consistent with complete objectivity in advising one's institution on the award of a half million dollar annual contract? There was only one conclusion: 'No way, Jose'!

There also are casual or uncompromising gifts which have little social significance – politicians shaking hands with strangers in a crowd, gratifying their own thirst for popularity by giving out moments of media-recognition in exchange. Others are: payment of unspecified 'tips' for small services rendered; giving anonymously to charities, etc. Also in this casual category is the 'give-away' information with which Industry floods doctors' offices. This 'give-away' (also called 'throw-away') material promotes the interests of Industry at so casual a level of gift-giving as to establish no relationship or exert undue influence.

Certainly, most professionals are well able to resist these influences, but at the same time it must also be admitted that there are many precedent examples of unethical behaviour in medicine, as in the worlds of business and politics. Clearly, the amount of money involved matters, as does the value of a gift. The situation warrants particular examination when the donor is very affluent and the recipient either relatively poor or relatively vulnerable to influence.

II. Where do conflicts of interest occur in relation to industry?

Physicians and medical researchers encounter ethical conflict where three sets of interests meet: their own, those of Industry, and those of patients or research subjects. These points of possible conflict are illustrated in Figure 1. It is, of course, impossible to delineate the whole of this complex relationship in a short treatise, but figure 1 is an attempt to systematize the areas of interaction.

The first four avenues of commercially sponsored activity are seen as affecting physicians and medical researchers attitudes via the institutions which serve them. In these four areas, influence from Industry is indirect, non-coercive and ethically acceptable, for the most part. For the sake of comparison with the remaining areas, these may be termed as Industry's support of the 'affective' or preparatory side of the practising physician or researcher. Activities numbered 5–8, in contrast, are areas in which the researcher or physician actually participates by directly using products or devices which are 'on the market' or being researched for efficacy and eventual licensure. This may be termed the 'effector' aspect of this subject.

First, – 'support of basic research'. This is best exemplified by the relationship established between Industry and Government. In the USA this is effected through Co-operative Research and Development Agreement Programs [7]. In Canada, there are joint ventures between the Medical Research Council and Industry [8] whereby industrial funds for areas of specific research are matched and distributed

94

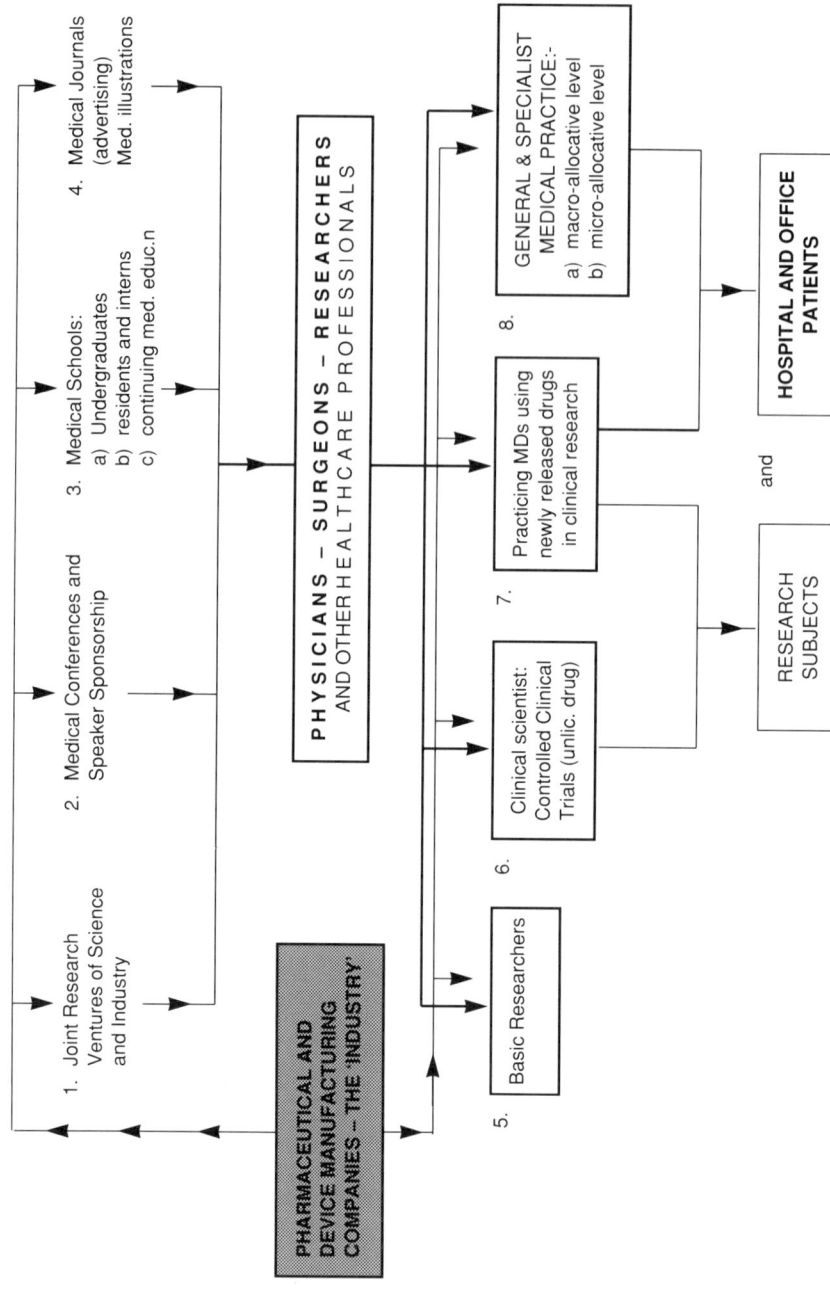

Figure 1. Eight points of interaction of Medical Science and Practice with 'Industry'.

by M.R.C. only if independent scientific peer review deems projects to merit funding. This type of joint activity may influence the independence of federal research but the mutual interests of government and researchers are balanced, and it is unlikely that researchers or research subjects would not be well protected from lack of ethical controls via IRBs and other review committees.

The Industry may also make major research contracts directly with University Departments to mutual advantage of each, without individual researchers being at risk of undesirable compromises.

Second, – 'support of professional organizations'. This is the sponsorship of specific speakers and holding of special symposia at medical professional association conferences or annual meetings. Of course, Industry selects which topics it will sponsor but the process is open and usually Industry does not pick the speaker. In another model Industry selects both speaker and topic for a sponsored tour, but even then the process is open and the speaker is not required to promote a given product, though the company's product will presumably be one of those mentioned as efficacious.

Third, – 'support the training process'. At the level of the medical schools and training institutions, Industry shows considerable interest in assisting impecunious undergraduates: to acquire equipment, including their traditional black bags; to learn about certain drugs from therapy sessions sponsored by a specific company; to help in funding interns' and residents' travel to scientific or medical meetings; and by providing special lectures for interns and residents (often in association with beer and pretzels, or even wine and cheese). There is no doubt that this has an influence on student and intern awareness of Industry and their products. In one review [6], residents deemed gifts or perquisites ('perks') worth over $100 as undesirable. They also questioned the value of allowing such contacts, in the first place.

At the post-graduate level or in Continuing Medical Education, University sponsored courses may fail to attract practitioners unless they associate with Industry, the latter often providing the lavish dinner or banquet.

Fourth, – 'facilitate learning about products in the journals' – through product advertising. Advertisements are displayed colourfully and dramatically. Advertisements no longer are confined to the front and back of journals. They are interwoven into the scientific pages. This would seem to be a form of influence which, though regrettable, is legitimate and non-coercive.

Fifth – 'help the basic researcher in the lab.' – This is the area where the basic researcher is *directly* helped by Industry. This may take the form of industry/researcher contract, directly solicited by either party, initially. Some contracts may circumvent the peer review system for research priorities. Care must be taken to have full disclosure of the 'deal' and to avoid unethical compromises which come from accepting disproportionate honoraria, etc. Purchasing stock in the company must be avoided as it smacks of 'insider trading'. For many such projects, because the research funding is provided by the Industry, the Research Ethics Board (REB) or Institutional Research Board (IRB) serves both for review of ethics as well as scientific merit, and unfortunate fact as they usually are competent only for the former function.

Sixth, – 'help the clinical trialist'. Industry's assistance is offered to those carrying out controlled clinical trials with promising new products, not yet licensed. Usually the agent is supplied free by the company and the protocol is often a joint composition by industry and researcher. The consent form may also reflect this mixture of concerns. Although protection of the research subject should be the most critical aspect, it sometimes takes second place to the interests of the company. Protection of the company from foreseeable risk, ensuring Industry's access to the data, and protection of Industry's copyrights and patent rights should not take precedence over the researcher's autonomy, research subjects' confidentiality and the process of fully informed consent. Therapy for the control group, for example, must be the best currently available, rather than another product of the same company which may not meet that criterion. Other questions which arise are: if a drug is successful, but expensive, will it subsequently be made available free of charge to the control group which helped to establish its efficacy? When trial 'B' elsewhere has established efficacy for drug X, which might imply that the current trial 'A' should be stopped inconclusively, will recruitment be continued in order to establish efficacy of X in trial 'A', too? In multi-centre trials, it is important that a professional group, not Industry, control the dynamics of the trial and evaluation of results – not the company – making them available to the company secondarily, even when the company is 'paying the shot'. In this category, also, the ethics review committee also frequently finds itself acting as the main institutional review for scientific merit – providing another ethical loophole. Seventh, – 'explore new products jointly' in marketing research, after licensure. New drugs are usually released before the following questions can be answered: How does the newly licensed product operate in the market place? What are the interactions with other drugs which will become apparent as the new drug is used more widely? What are the unanticipated drug complications not revealed in the pre-licensure trials? What are the long-term (2 year, 5 year) effects? Market research to provide such answers is very important but faces such ethical hazards as: is payment to the clinician or his/her assistants based on numbers of patients recruited ethically acceptable? It should not be. The principles to be adopted by market researchers are: rewards should be discussed and settled ahead of time and be proportionate to time invested at predetermined levels of expertise; the need must be recognised for full disclosure to directors, colleagues and research subjects; subjects should not be paid except for expenses, loss of income, etc.; gifts should not be accepted; collaborating physicians should participate both in analysis of data and its publication. And, most importantly, patients must be fully informed that they are in a research study to which they are required to give informed consent, even though the drug is already approved. As such studies may emanate from physicians' offices, and not come before an institutional ethics review board, the practitioner may unwittingly involved in unconsented research.

Eighth, – 'shopping in the drug and device bazaar'. This is the largest area of all: the interaction between the practising physician and products of established value (drugs or devices) and already widely used in 'the market'. Here the emphasis is on making physicians familiar with drugs by 'brand' names which then become part of their regular armamentarium, to the exclusion of other products with similar or identical actions. Information about the new agent is passed to the busy practitioner by the company's PRs, together with various memory prompts and marketing aids. A veritable slurry of brand-name marked desk pads, calendars, rulers, pens and minor items of medical equipment flows across the practitioner's desk on its way to the trash can though much, it must be admitted, also spends time in white-coat pocket or on a shelf or desk where they imprint the mind of the practitioner with biased (though not necessarily false) information. Many practitioners obtain updating on pharmacology and therapeutics, by this route – hopefully not exclusively so.

A special case is devices. These are usually external and do not have to face the same rigorous pre-market licensure process as do drugs. Controlled trial evidence for efficacy or effectiveness is usually not required before being registered as safe even though devices such as lithotripters are directly invasive of tissues (though not of the skin) and also very costly [9]. Dialysers for hemodialysis are also included in this category.

Whereas Figure 1 purports to cover many areas where ethical conflict may arise between the interests of industry, practitioners, researchers, research subjects and patients, it does not indicate the nature of the conflict and the ethical principles involved. These are considered, below.

III. Ethical principles and rules involved in interactions with industry

These include:

1. *Beneficence in finding new ways of treating disease.* This ethical principle is shared by both the health care professions and Industry. At the highest level of abstraction, both are working for the good of society. Both the physician's personal income and industrial profits are instrumental to this good. The essential difference is that physicians also have a strong duty to protect patients from harm – nonmaleficence – and to promote their patients' interests, even in preference to their own (provided the two sets are not in moral conflict) [10], whereas Industry's interests are those of 'company profit through competition'. Benefit to patients is incidental to successful business competition.

2. *Autonomy of drug firms – in a private enterprise capitalist system.* This social ethic is strongly defended in our capitalistic political philosophy. We may have to lay down rules and guidelines within which such autonomy is controlled but,

broadly speaking, we want to guard the right of those in Industry to pursue their profit-seeking ends with little restraint, no more than is necessary to protect professional responsibility for the public good. It should not be forgotten that over 90% of new drugs emanate from the research investment of the pharmaceutical industry, and no device would be safe without supervised manufacture to pre-set industrial standards.

3. *Autonomy of physicians and researchers – academic and professional freedom.* Our society recognizes that individual health care professionals (physicians and researchers) should have the freedom to do what they want provided it is within the law and the ethical guidelines of their profession. Nevertheless, there are obvious risks to public good and ethics from uncontrolled scientific exploitation in such areas as genetic engineering and the new reproductive technologies. There is urgent need for societal guidelines in such areas, where the issue is one of research legitimacy, not one of research process. Within these critically important domains, we need societal limits for scientific exploration based on moral, philosophical, theological and religious agreement – not a simple matter for a pluralistic liberal democratic society. Freedom for health care professionals to work with Industry within ethical boundaries is but a part of that larger societal decision.

4. *Patients' autonomy: The right to choose between all treatment options on the basis of totally unbiased information.* In renal failure, Industry's profit-driven promotion of one treatment modality – dialysis – is possible cause for compromise of patients' treatment options. Some physicians become biased in one direction or another in the choice of drugs, in the choice of dialysis modalities (home dialysis vs in-centre), as well as in the wider choice between dialysis and transplantation. Those who believe that some nephrologists have been unduly influenced towards the dialysis modality, and therefore do not present the option of transplantation in a fair light, term these patients as being 'trapped in dialysis'[11]. In Europe, for example, transplanted patients per million of population (pmp) vary from 61 and 109 in Italy and Spain to 252 and 226 in Norway and Sweden, though the numbers on chronic renal failure management for these 4 countries is comparable (330, 351, 301 and 395 pmp, respectively) [12]. Also, only one quarter of dialysis patients were reported as being listed for renal transplantation though many believe that this should be in the range of 50% (even when the aging of patients receiving renal failure management is taken into account).

The role of the dialysis Industry in shaping physicians' opinions on the renal transplantation option is quite unknown, of course. But research on the question is needed in order to determine reasons for these wide range of transplantation practices in managing chronic renal failure. Data for similar influences in the USA is less available, but also needs to be researched; the variation in renal cadaver donor rates per million population could have many contributing factors.

5. *Issues of distributive justice.* The issue of 'trapped in dialysis' is not only an issue of patient autonomy but also distributive justice. Dialysis is very costly; transplantation (though not proven beyond all doubt to give longer life) is unquestionably more cost effective. However, the role of Industry in this issue, as mentioned above, is not clear.

The most significant resource allocation issue in the interaction between health care and Industry concerns costly brand-name drugs in comparison with less expensive generic products. Physicians have a duty to study this area, by being aware of relative costs and valid differences. Professional organizations also have a duty to publicise the economic facts of prescribing habits. There is no doubt that much cost could be saved to government health care systems by carefully controlling the freedom to prescribe brand-name products when comparable generic products are available. At the same time, the issue is not a simple one. A good habit for physicians would be only to use generic names whenever possible, both in parlance and prescribing, though this policy is by no means easy to carry out as the full force of the PRs is against it.

IV. What are the safeguards? Where are the solutions?

As already mentioned, most individuals are able to resist, but the mechanisms of resistance involve: i) having enough time to think about the issue, ii) having enough alternative drug or device information, which is unbiased by commercial interests, flowing through professional channels of communication, and iii) being able to maintain a valid foundation of basic knowledge into which the new drug and device information may be absorbed. For many physicians, in busy practice (see 8 b) in Figure 1), these three defense systems are insufficient leading to undue influence from the PRs. This influence of PRs may be subtly reinforced by their invitation to Industry-sponsored educational symposia or post-graduate events (see area 2 and 3 b) in Figure 1).

Ways in which these tendencies might be countered at the micro-economic level include professionally controlled and planned post-graduate medical education, attendance at which should probably should be mandated by licensing colleges. Legitimate scepticism would lead to less prescribing. Attention to relative costs would lead to increased cost effectiveness. Computerized diskettes for use by physicians in the office, regularly updated, might wrest control of prescribing habits back into the hands of the professionals from their commercial advisors.

In the research field, joint ventures of the type indicated in area 1 in Figure 1, is probably the best way to go. At the macro-economic level, special arrangements between institutions and industry are increasing in number and importance. Protection from undue influence or compromise in this area must come through the principle of full disclosure of all special arrangements and wide discussion of the implications, in advance.

100

As with most problems, to dissect it for inspection may also be of critical importance in enabling individuals to become more alert to the influences which are playing upon them. This is the primary aim of this chapter.

References

1. Royal College of Physicians. The relationship between physicians and the pharmaceutical industry. J R Coll Phys Lond 1986; 20: 235–42.
2. American College of Physicians. Physicians and the pharmaceutical industry. Ann Intern Med 1990; 112: 624–6.
3. Canadian Psychiatric Association Guidelines in Relating to the Pharmaceutical Industry. Can J Psychiat 1987; 32: 476–80.
4. Palea J. NIH grapples with conflict of interest. Science 1989; 245: 23.
5. Conflicts of Interest in Medical Center/Industry Research Relationships. Council report. JAMA 1990; 263: 2790–3.
6. McKinney WP, Schiedermayer DL, Lurie D et al. Attitudes of internal medicine faculty and residents toward professional interactions with pharmaceutical sales representatives. JAMA 1990; 264: 1693–7.
7. Culliton BJ NIH, Inc: the CRADA boom. Science 1989; 245: 1034–6.
8. University-Industry Grants and Awards Guide, 1990/91. Ministry of Supply and Services, Canada 1990: Cat. no. MR2-2/1991.
9. Wiser LC, Plain RHM, Dossetor JB. Kidney stones and lithotripters: Critical analysis of the introduction of extracorporeal shock wave lithotripsy (ESWL) into Canada. Can Med Assoc J 1990; 143: 1299–1303.
10. Pellegrino ED. The physician as gatekeeper (chapter 14) In Pellegrino ED, Thomasma DC (eds.): For the patient's good: the restoration of beneficence in health care O.U.P.; 1989.
11. See discussion in Proceedings of First Joint Conference (E.S.O.T. and E.D.T.A.) on Ethics, Justice and Commerce in Organ Replacement Therapy. (Munich, 1990, Springer Verlag – in press).
12. Combined Report on Regular Dialysis and Transplantation in Europe, XIX, 1988. Nephrology, dialysis and transplantation 1989; 4 (supplement 4): 5–40.

PART THREE

Stopping treatment

8. Practical aspects of stopping dialysis and cultural differences

CARL M. KJELLSTRAND

Stopping dialysis, as a cause of death is common, particularly in North America. In the USA it is now the third most common cause of death in dialysis patients, and in Canada the second most common cause, after vascular deaths, as illustrated in Figure 1.

When dialysis is stopped the patient who needs it will invariably die. In 155 dialysis patients, we studied the consequences of stopping dialysis. Death occurred after a mean of 8.1 days (range 1–28 days) [1]. The number of days from the last dialysis to the death of each patient is shown in Figure 2. Port and co-workers doing a similar analysis in 282 patients concluded that it took somewhat longer

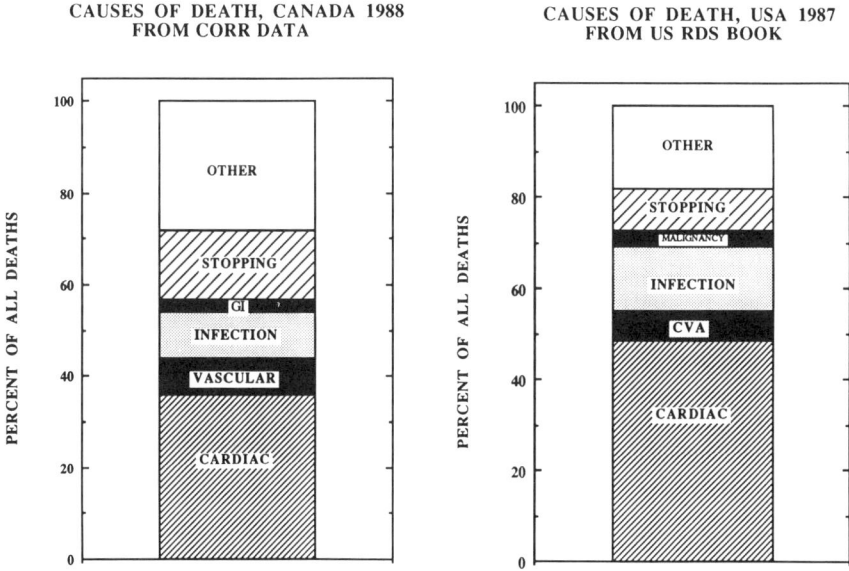

Figure 1. Causes of death in USA and Canada in the late 1980s.
In Canada, stopping dialysis is the second most common cause of death, in the USA it is the third.
CORR = Canadian Organ Replacement Registry. RDS = Renal Data System

103

C. M. Kjellstrand and J. B. Dossetor (eds): Ethical Problems in Dialysis and Transplantation, 103–116.
© 1992 *Kluwer Academic Publishers. Printed in the Netherlands.*

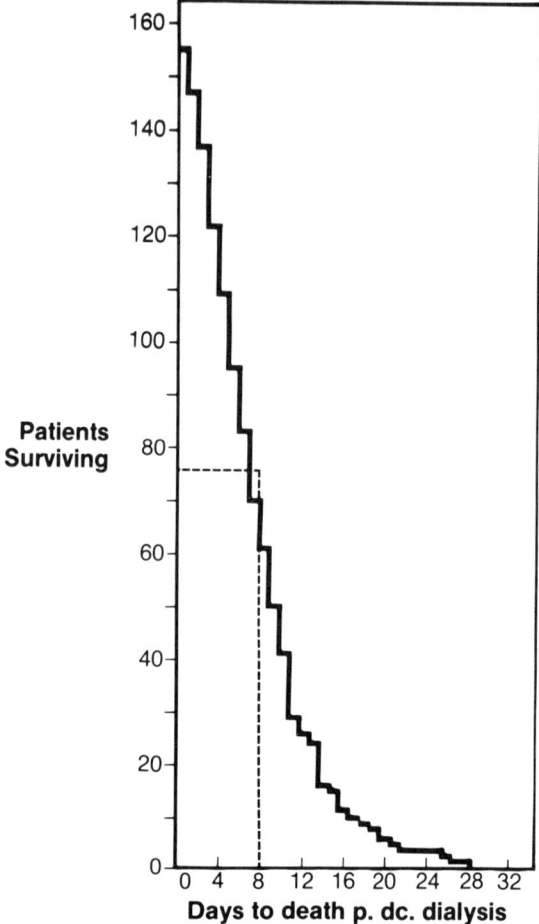

Figure 2. Time to death after last dialysis, in 155 patients who stopped dialysis.

time, about 10 days [2]. One reason for the difference may be that CAPD patients have better preserved renal function.

The general practical outline to stopping dialysis is presented in Table I [3].

Table I. The analysis of stopping dialysis

PLANE I – ETHICAL ANALYSIS
---

1. *ETHICAL FRAMEWORK* – KANTIAN DEONTOLOGY

BENEFICENCE	– ('Sanctity of Life')
NONMALEFICENCE	– Do Not Cause Suffering
AUTONOMY	– Respect Dignity and Difference

2. *INTELLECTUAL/EMOTIONAL ANALYSIS* – EXISTENTIALISM

Weigh Burden vs Benefit: Suffering vs. Lifegain
Non-maleficence and Autonomy vs Beneficence

3. *PRACTICAL ANALYSIS CONSEQUENCE*: – CLASSICAL UTILITARIANISM

What are the Alternatives?

ACT	*CONSEQUENCES*
Do Everything	Analyze
Change Course	and
Do Less	Predict
Stop Everything	

PLANE II – PRACTICAL ANALYSIS
---

1. MEDICAL ASPECTS: Disease Understood

Prognosis Known
Maximal Care Tried
Do Experts Agree

2. WHY DO YOU WANT TO STOP:

Patient's Best Interest
Family Desperate
Friends Squeamish
Team Discouraged
You Depressed and Tired

3. MAKING THE DECISION

Be Prepared
DISCUSS-LISTEN-DOCUMENT

4. UNSOLVABLES:

Patient Undecided or Periodically lucid.
Family Feuds

5. WHAT DO YOU PLAN TO DO:

DO NOT KILL
Do Not Practice Medical Scrupulosity

PLANE III – AFTER DISCONTINUATION
---

1. AFTER STOPPING – Visit Patient   – Do no bloodsamples,

– Watch and prevent pulmonary edema

2. AFTER PATIENT IS DEAD

– Follow up with family
– Consequences for family

Although the table presents the approach in logical stepwise fashion on three planes, in fact these considerations are simultaneously considered and intertwined.

I. Plane I – Ethical analysis

Ethical principles which bear on stopping life support will be discussed in detail in Chapter 11. Using these principles, three approaches to ethics analysis are suggested.

The first is Kantian deontology. There is an apparent inflexibility when staunch right-to-life arguments are applied in such a way that sanctity of life trumps all other duties, and prohibits all thought of termination of life-sustaining treatment. However, most physicians do not hold that beneficence is captured by absolute sanctity of life arguments. They also do not subscribe to a view that beneficence always takes priority over duties to avoid maleficence or promote patient autonomy. For them, the 'categorical imperative' (or unconditional principle that can be universally applied) becomes 'physician have obligations to promote patients' autonomy and their best interests', not 'physicians are always obliged to preserve life under all conceivable conditions.' Once this flexibility is introduced and understood, the objection that deontologic analysis can be too rigid, even cruel, in medical decision-making is negated.

The second analytic approach is existentialist. It is clear that only competent patients can quantitate burdens and benefits and then do the balancing that results in a decision, using whatever basis for judgement that seems right for them, as individuals. If the patient is incompetent, close relatives and friends must judge what the patient would have wished to be done. We have previously shown, that the decision made by competent patients is identical to that made by physicians and families on behalf of the incompetent patient [4]. Thus, the argument that no-one can decide for someone else that it is better to be dead, is not correct. On the contrary, one can turn the tables and ask why one should force an incompetent patient to accept a treatment that a competent patient would not accept. After all, an incompetent patient no longer can appreciate the benefits and purpose of dialysis and thus suffers more than a competent patient who can still hopes for success or improvement. In such an analysis, one weighs non-maleficence and autonomy versus beneficence, here understood as sanctity of life. For the incompetent, the family and physician consider suffering and potential survival time and weigh these against each other to finally decide whether treatment should be continued or stopped. These family-physician considerations are similar to the Catholic church's consideration of extraordinary treatment where burdens against benefits are weighed [5]. Obviously if patients are competent they do this weighing, using clear and accurate facts from their physicians, and emotional support from family, treatment team, physician and clergyman. An important duty here is for the physician to rule out underlying psychiatric abnormality which might induce the patient give up too early, and one must be sure that the patient has no treatable somatic complication which might tip the balance in favour of stopping treatment.

The third analytic approach is to perform an utilitarian analysis. One considers all possible treatment alternatives and tries to foresee positive and negative consequences and choose the course which maximises benefit. Should one continue to do everything because there is a reasonable chance of improvement? Would shorter treatment times allow more freedom for the patient? Would dialysis away at a vacation facility be of help? Should one stop everything and let a patient die? Should one change course, is another dialysis method or dialysis place possible and would such a change help the patient? Would CAPD at home be more suitable for the in-centre patient, or would the reverse be true? Would it be better to stop treatment at home and transfer to in-centre to get the emotional support from the hospital team of caregivers?

In one article, it was more common for home dialysis patients than in-centre patients to stop treatment when there was no medical reason to do so [6]. We speculated that at home, the patient was the only sick person with nobody but close family members on whom to vent anger and frustration, and was used to making important medical decisions alone. But the underlying equation was to maximize utility or most good for the patient – an exercise in act utilitarianism.

II. Plane II – Practical analysis

Several medical aspects need consideration. Is the disease and its prognosis known and understood? The confusional dementia secondary to an acute illness such as septicemia in al old patient is different from the relentless downward course of dialysis dementia at the end-stage of aluminium intoxication or that secondary to many strokes. An endogenous depression may be treatable by antidepressants. Reactive depression secondary to a transient mishap in personal life is different from the truly miserable situation of the diabetic patient who progressively loses vision and then limbs through amputation. Kaye and associates have analyzed and defined the instances when one need not heed patients' wishes to stop treatment in order to allow time to overcome such transient setbacks [7].

Another important aspect is to be sure one has tried available therapy to the fullest extent. The Australian Anaesthesiology Association suggests employing maximal therapy for at least three weeks before one decides to withdraw it. In general, it appears unwise to discontinue chronic dialysis under the pressure of acute situations. Finally, it is important to make sure that necessary consultation has taken place, and that the consultants are in agreement that the situation is hopeless. Clearly, one should not stop therapy if a neurologist asks for a few more days to evaluate progress or to determine the irreversibility of dementia or cerebral damage caused by a stroke.

The second step in the common sense practical analysis is to reflect on why one is agreeing with a patient's wish to stop dialysis. Is it really in the patient's best interest? Is the situation truly hopeless? Is it really correct that conditions can only worsen. Are there other factors operating? Is the family desperate because things are going too slowly? Are the friends squeamish because of tubes, a respirator or temporary absence of control of bodily functions? Is the team of immediate care givers discouraged and demoralized? Have all relevant consultations been obtained?

In general, it appears that nurses tend to give up earlier than physicians. They are so much closer to the suffering, they see the patient continually. Physicians, on the contrary, are more remote from the daily struggle and perhaps, therefore, tend to give up too late. Maybe these different points of view create a healthy tension in the team's view of the patient's situation and perhaps results in 'just enough care given.' Is the doctor recommending termination of treatment because he/she is depressed and tired of seeing the patient day after day? Is frustration at the dubious possibility of a solution in the foreseeable future unduly influencing judgement? When considering all these conflicting interests and wishes, it is obvious that the only valid decision is one which reflects the patient's wishes or, if the patient has lost capacity, the patient's best interests.

Several points need to be made concerning the actual decision to terminate treatment. First, one must be prepared to anticipate this possibility and discuss it frankly and openly, yet with sensitivity, with both patient and family earlier on in treatment, even before dialysis becomes necessary and again after completing several months of dialysis. This is the area of advance treatment directives. Questions of death, dying, and withdrawal of treatment are always difficult for physicians; they may judge them threatening and frightening to patients. Studies have shown that the opposite appears to be true. Bernard Lo, discussing the use of antibiotics, nasogastric feeding, feeding tubes and use of respirators with a group of gravely ill patients with heart conditions and cancer, found that 68% of these patients wished to have such discussions with physicians and that most of them wished the physician to originate the discussion [8]. In actuality, only 6% had discussed life-sustaining treatment with a physician. When asked how the patients feel after this discussion, a questionnaire stated that 71% felt much better and that they had some control over these things, 53% felt relieved, and 53% felt cared for. Twenty-two percent said that they felt nervous about the discussion, 16% felt sad, and 6% felt like they wanted to give up. All in all, it appears clear that most patients want to have such discussion. Certainly, knowledge about the patient's wishes will considerably ease the decision making later on, should the patient become incompetent. This is the objective sought by all forms of advance treatment directives.

When patients are making decisions to discontinue treatment three things are important for the caregivers:

1. Be open about details and discuss them.
2. Listen carefully to what different family members and other members of the

team have to say. Ask them outright what they think about the situation, and understand that they often may have difficulty expressing an opposing view.

3. In case disagreements should arise in the future, the discussion must be carefully documented in the chart.

There are also instances where patient's decision to stop treatment must not be accepted – must be resisted. One is in the periodically undecided patient who may decide to stop treatment one day and continue treatment another. If so, one obviously proceeds until the patient had a prolonged period of lucidity and clarity and is capable of making a conclusive decision. The other outcome is when the patient becomes definitely incompetent. In that situation, the decision devolves onto family and caregivers, and if the family feuds over the decision, one has to continue treatment. When encountering such situations, the family should be told that their decision should be unanimous. If they are presently unable to reach a decision, they need to contemplate their positions, consider whether they need more medical information and whether they should confer with others, family friends or advisors or spiritual leaders for guidance. After a suitable period one can again bring up the question.

Consider carefully analgesics, fluid management and sedatives, but do not kill the patient. Only the Netherlands condones active killing of patients [9]. Doing so in any other country would almost certainly lead to a murder charge. On the other hand, one must not practice what the Catholic church calls medical scrupulosity, that is, the using of technology simply because it is there; that is a sin. The moral and humane consequences of the technologies must be considered.

III. Awaiting death

There are certain practical aspects in dealing with a patient who has decided to discontinue treatment and is waiting for death. The first is to warn the family that death may be a long time in coming, perhaps up to a month, so that they do not necessarily focus on the mean time of approximately one week. Secondly, they should be told that death in uremia is a comfortable death. The patient becomes increasingly lethargic and is usually found dead in bed, probably due to cardiac arrest secondary to hyperkalemia. However, progressive pulmonary edema leads to a horrible death, therefore fluid and sodium restriction needs to be maintained. Should fluid overload occur, oral or rectal Sorbitol can be used, or the patient can undergo ultrafiltration without dialysis. All other restrictions should be lifted.

One should not order any blood samples or absurd situations may arise, such as being called at night, or even worse having another on-call physician being asked to decide whether to treat hyperkalemia in the dying patient. Doing tests will indicate problems for which one would not contemplate doing anything. This is an unnecessary strain on everybody and a waste of resources. Do not do them!

However, patients awaiting death should be visited daily and contact should be maintained with their families. Listening to the chest, although it may appear an act of futility to the physician, is an act of kindness to the patient that tells him he has not been abandoned, and it eases the concern of the family that nobody cares, any more.

Finally, there are two aspects to take care of, even after the patient has died. Some people have suggested a follow-up visit with the family, so that questions they are pondering may be answered, and therefore their grief and uncertainty diminished [10, 11]. The second matter concerns preventing harms to the survivors, particularly if the patient was incompetent and the decision to discontinue was made by close family members with the caregivers. Deciding that the loved family member would be better off dead was obviously a momentous decision. Questions have been raised as to whether such a situation can do permanent harm to a family. Two teams have studied this. Walwork and associates [12] compared social functioning and grieving in families who had decided to stop respirator and life support of newborn babies to similar factors in families where the newborn baby had died while still on life support. There was no difference in grieving or social functioning between these two groups of families one year after the decision had been made. Roberts and co-workers wrote to 144 family members of dialysis patients who had died by withdrawal of treatment [13]. In general, the family members felt no particular anger for having participated in the decision, and felt it had not disturbed their peace of mind. They were generous in praising nurses, physicians, residents, social workers and chaplains as being helpful both in making the decision and in supporting them after the decision. They felt that physician and residents were the most helpful in making the decision and that social workers and nurses were the ones who supported them afterwards. They were most troubled in the cases where the patient had had no medical reason to withdraw but had done so only for reasons of stress, a situation most often occurring when patients withdraw treatment at home [6]. In answers to open ended questions, relatives were somewhat disappointed that physicians were so unwilling to talk to them about discontinuation of treatment, and suspected that physicians were overly optimistic and continued treatment for too long. They wished for more openness and truthfulness. No long term psychological harm seems to have come to relatives and family because of their involvement in the decision.

IV. Cultural differences

There are great differences between different geographical regions in the incidence rates of suicide and stopping dialysis. Thus, stopping treatment or committing suicide in North America appears to be three times as common as in Europe and six times as common as in Japan.

Within the United States there are marked differences in the rate of stopping

MICHIGAN DIALYSIS REGISTRY 1982 - 84

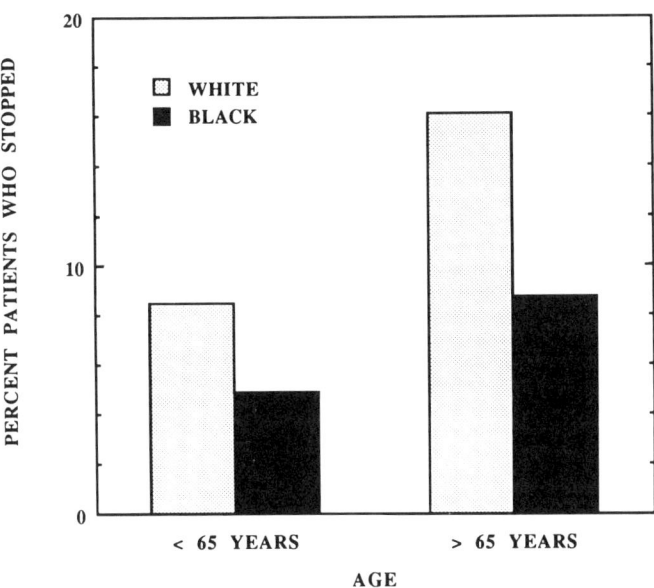

Figure 3. Stopping dialysis is twice as common among whites as among black patients [2].

treatment, depending on race. Thus, in a review of the Michigan Dialysis Registry, Port et al. [2] found that stopping treatment was twice as common among whites as among blacks (Figure 3). One can only speculate about the reasons. Black patients seem to be more eager to get their older family members on dialysis. Kjellstrand and Logan found that the incidence of starting dialysis in blacks over the age of 64 years was twice that of whites when comparing those who choose to start dialysis to those who died of chronic kidney failure. The higher incidence of kidney failure in blacks thus does not explain this difference [14]. Perhaps then this special care that black patients want to give their elderly is also reflected when the possibility of stopping treatment comes up. The other problem may be one of communication. Most physicians doing dialysis are white and perhaps communication problems exist more often between the white physicians and black patients [15]. Dr Callender, a black transplant physician himself, has commented on the superstition, lack of education, and general distrust that black patients have of physicians [16, 17].

Superficially, even more profound differences can be found between Western Europe and North America. In Figure 4 are plotted data from Europe and Minnesota that are quite similar to that in USA and Canada [1, 18]. While almost 9% of patients in Minnesota ultimately due because dialysis was stopped, this is true for only 3.1% of patients in Europe. However, when one examines age distri-

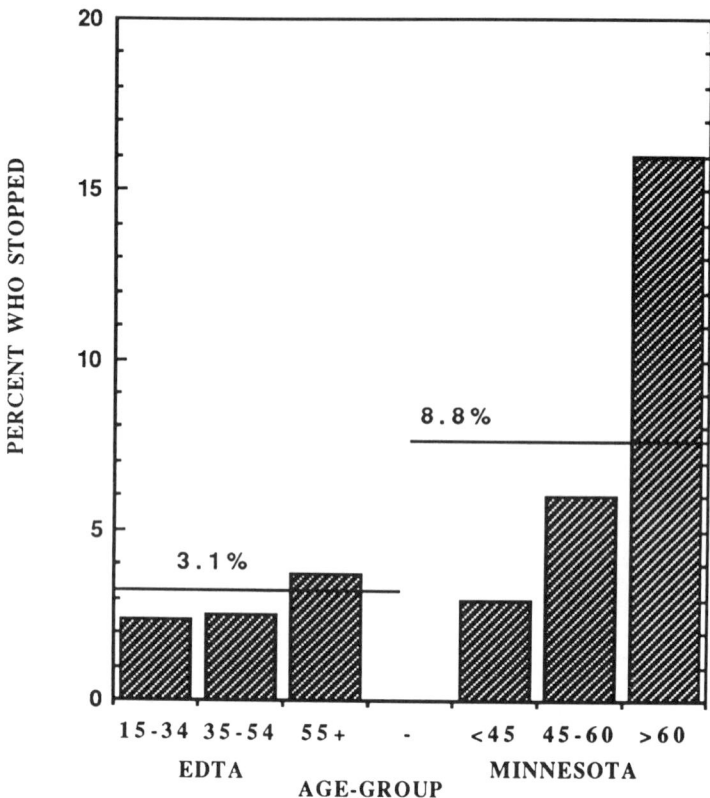

Figure 4. Stopping dialysis, a comparison of European and Minnesota Data. Overall stopping is three times as common in Minnesota, but part of this explanation may be that the US patients are older and more sick than European patients.

bution, a startling difference is seen with older patients. In Europe these patients are not directly comparable because of different age limits. Perhaps the reason for the threefold difference in stopping treatment is that, in the United States, many more elderly patients are started on dialysis. This group have a particularly high rate of discontinuation of treatment, and in these elderly patients pre-existing disease is particularly common. It has been shown that pre-existing diseases are much more common among those patients who ultimately stop treatment (Figure 5).

Perhaps there is also a difference of attitude. In general, the European system appears more paternalistic than that in North America. Wehle and Ahlmén analyzing the pattern of stopping in Sweden, comment that 'the ultimate decision has to be made by the Head of the Department' [19]. This indicates a more hierarchical type of decision-making than in North America where the decision is more a per-

PRE-EXISTING DISEASES

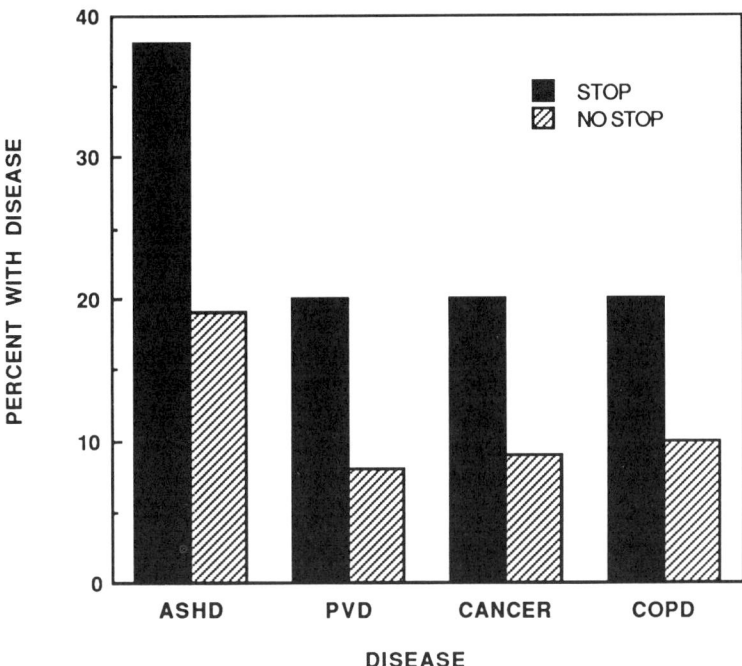

Figure 5. Stopping treatment as a cause of death, and pre-existing disease in Minnesota. Other serious diseases at start of dialysis are twice as common in patients who die from stopping dialysis as in the patients who do not stop therapy.

sonal one, made between patient, physician and other caregivers especially nurses rather than by an official administrative physician, who may not know the patient well.

There are also some consequences of this difference in approach. In Europe, acute acts of deliberate suicide among dialysis patients are twice as common as in Minnesota (Figure 6). Perhaps desperate patients in Europe are more likely to end their lives in a violent fashion because bureaucratic physicians in Europe are less responsive to their needs than the more personal treatment team would be in North America.

In Japan the pattern of stopping dialysis is entirely different from that in Europe and North America (Figure 7). While stopping treatment and committing suicide shows a marked increase with age both in Europe and in North America (Figure 4), the reverse is true in Japan. Five percent of patients in Japan below the age of 30 end their lives by terminating therapy or committing suicide and this figure falls to less than 1% in patients over the age of 60 years. Thus, as a percentage of death, actually ending treatment or committing suicide is not more common in young

114

SUICIDE, PERCENT

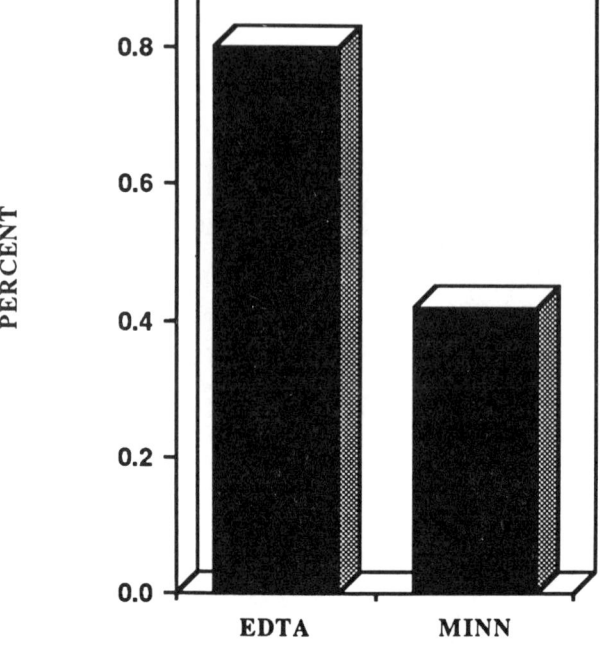

Figure 6. Suicide is twice as common in dialysis patients in Europe as in Minnesota.

patients in Europe and USA than in Japan, but in the patient above age 60 stopping therapy is 30 times more common in USA than it is in Japan. Once can only specu-late over the reasons. Perhaps the young patients in Japan feel particularly desper-ate as almost no transplants are done in this country, and it has been shown that it is the young who are particularly fervent about wishing to be transplanted, while this wish declines steeply with age [20]. Patients in Europe or North America who are young can look forward almost with certainty to receiving a transplant. This is not the case in Japan. However, this does not explain the markedly low incidence of discontinuation of treatment and committing suicide in the old Japanese patients. Our understanding is that any prohibition against suicide can not explain this differ-ence as suicide as a solution to a difficult personal situation appears to be more acceptable to the Japanese than to almost any other culture. Perhaps it has to do with a general attitude to getting old. Clearly Western societies adulate the young

DATA FROM THE 1986 JAPANESE DIALYSIS REGISTRY

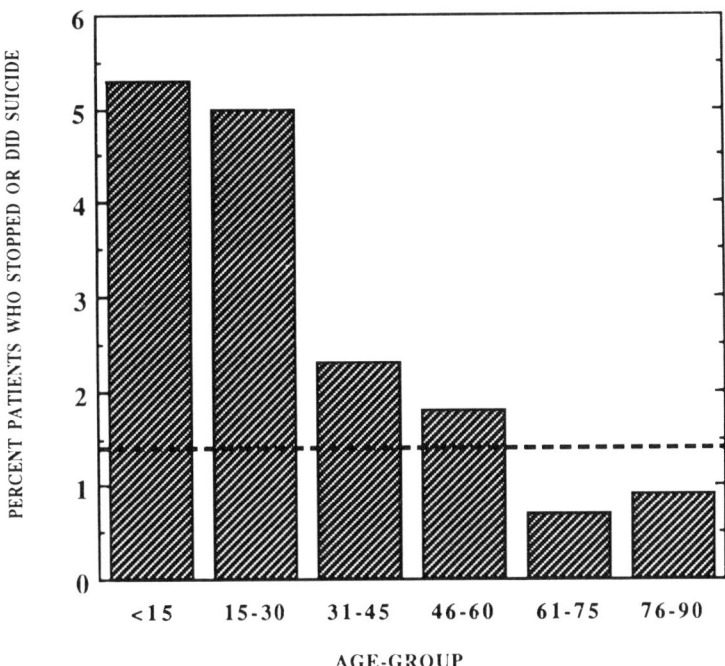

Figure 7. Stopping treatment and committing suicide as causes of death of dialysis patients in Japan. In Japan, contrary to USA and Europe, it is the young who stop treatment or commit suicide, not the old.

and forget the old, but the reverse is true in Japan. To be old in Japan is to be considered not only wise, but to be a repository of knowledge, and to have the power of judgement that is admired and utilized and this may make the older Japanese patients feel a better sense of worth.

References

1. Neu S. Kjellstrand CM. Stopping long-term dialysis. An empirical study of withdrawal of life-supporting treatment. N. Engl J Med 1986; 314: 14–20.
2. Port FK, Wolfe RA, Hawthorne VM *et al.* Ferguson CW. Discontinuation of dialysis therapy as a cause of death. Am J Neph 1989 9: 145–9.
3. Kjellstrand CM. Giving life – giving death. Ethical problems with high technology medicine. Ph.D. Thesis. Karolinska Institute, Stockholm 1988 and Acta Medica Scandinavica Supplementum 1988; Suppl 725.
4. Munoz JE, Kjellstrand CM. Withdrawing life support: do families and physicians decide as patients do? Nephron 1988; 48: 201–5.

5. Sacred Congregation for the Doctrine of the Faith. Declaration on Euthanasia Ottawa, Ontario, Publication Service, Canadian Conference of Catholic Bishops 1980.
6. Roberts J, Kjellstrand CM. Choosing death: Withdrawal without medical reason from chronic dialysis. Acta Med Scand 1988; 223: 181–6.
7. Kaye M, Bourgouin P, Low G. Physicians' non-compliance with patients' refusal of life-sustaining treatment. Am J Nephrol 1987; 7: 304–12.
8. Lo B, McLeod GA, Saika G. Patient attitudes to discussing life-sustaining treatment. Arch Intern Med 1986; 146: 1613–5.
9. Pence GE. Do not go slowly into that dark night: mercy killing in Holland. Am J Med 1988; 84: 139–41.
10. Sandbert S, Holm L, Enger E. Veilednings – og omsorgsbehov hos etterlatte. Tidskr Nor Lœgeforen 1985; 105: 1412–5.
11. Tolle S, Bascom PB, Hickam DH et al. Communication between physicians and surviving spouses following patient death. J Gen Intern Med 1986; 1: 309 –14.
12. Walwork E, Ellison PH. Follow up of families of neonates in whom life support was withdrawn. Clin Ped 1985; 24: 14–20.
13. Roberts J, Snyder R, Kjellstrand CM. Withdrawal of life support – The survivors. Acta Med Scand, 1988; 224: 141–8.
14. Kjellstrand CM, Logan G. Racial, sexual and age inequalities in chronic dialysis. Nephron 1987; 45: 257–63.
15. Kjellstrand CM, Racial, sexual and age inequalities in renal transplantation. Arch Intern Med 1988; 148: 1305–9.
16. Callender CO. Organ donation in blacks: a community approach. Transpl Proceed 1987; 19: 1551–4.
17. Callender CO. Organ donation in the black population: where do we go from here: Transpl Proceed 1987; 19, suppl 2: 36–40.
18. Combined report on regular dialysis and transplantation in Europe 1979. In Robinson BHB, Hawkins JB (eds): Proceedings of the European dialysis and transplant association, Vol. 17. Pitman Medical Limited: London 1980.
19. Wehle B, Ahlmén J. Prudent withdrawal of chronic dialysis treatment. Scand J Urol Nephrol Suppl 1990; 131: 47–8.
20. Kjellstrand CM, Lins LE, Ericson F et al. On the wish for renal transplantation. Transactions ASAIO 1989; 35: 619–21.

9. Religious aspects of stopping treatment

MICHAEL KAYE

It is one of the paradoxes of history that believers in Judaism, Christianity or Islam have spent so much effort, time and blood in fighting among themselves and with each other yet there is so much that is common and jointly held by each of the three great monotheistic religions. All share the view of a single Deity who created the world and everything within it and at the centre of this creation is mankind, made in the image and likeness of the Creator. As each of these religious traditions developed, first Judaism, then Christianity and subsequently Islam, so each faith built on what had existed previously but added new insights and doctrines of its own. Without intending to trivialize the many differences between these three faiths, from a twentieth century secular viewpoint, their unity in a belief in a divine Being, in man's intimate relation to that Being and his purpose on earth to serve the Divine, provides far more apparent similarity than diversity.

It is against this framework, that the practicalities of ethical decision making, as it pertains to cessation of dialysis, require consideration. Excluded will be those whose acceptance of their religious tradition is nominal only and who do not consider themselves as, in any way, bound by its precepts. The 'Christian' who is baptized, married and who will be buried by the Church but whose contact is limited to such rituals, is unlikely to seriously attempt to follow or be guided by the Church's moral and ethical teaching. While the individual, as part of a social group, may well follow certain practices and agree with certain views, this is more a form of group behaviour than a personal testimony arising from strong personal religious views. Such individuals – very many in the West – will not be the primary subjects of this chapter. Rather, the religious motivations of those for whom their beliefs form an important, often major place in their daily life, will be considered when the issue of discontinuation of dialysis arises.

Within the views of Judaism, Christianity and Islam, mankind is not alone, not a solitary agent, not an individual adrift in an ocean with only his own resources and responsibilities but instead is tied, related, serving something wholly other, outside of the person and bearing a special relation to him or her. As a result, life has a unique value and significance. It is not freely given or taken but instead carries a unique importance because the giver and supporter of that life is none other than the Divine Being. The earthly journey is not an enterprise undertaken without

117

C. M. Kjellstrand and J. B. Dossetor (eds): Ethical Problems in Dialysis and Transplantation, 117–125.
© 1992 *Kluwer Academic Publishers. Printed in the Netherlands.*

thought to any ultimate meaning or significance. On the contrary, it is an event for which the individual is and will be held accountable. That person and group, with whom they associate, is compelled to consider standards for conduct and thought which have originated in the sacred words and books, are embedded in tradition and have survived through the centuries. From this basic rationale, the developments in biomedical ethics related to termination of life support must be viewed and will be arranged in order of increasing latitude of individual opinion and autonomy.

I. Islam

The Holy book, the Quran and the law, or Shari'a, form the basis for all behaviour. Man is the Divine viceregent [1] or deputy here and now, and the preservation, conduct and enhancement of life on earth are paramount. Hence abortion is restricted and suicide and euthanasia are completely forbidden [2]. The time of death is dependent on the will of Allah [3] and man

has no right to terminate life except for judicial reasons. [4]

Therefore, even with the most remote possibility of recovery, continuation of life support remains justified in Islamic thought. However, where any chance of recovery is absent, and life support is only prolonging the inevitability of death, there appears to be general agreement that it can be discontinued [5, 6]. Death, if and when it occurs, is then determined by Allah [7]. Medical judgement is therefore necessary and differences of opinion may be present as to whether any possibility of recovery exists. In such circumstances, life support would be continued. As indicated, with the conscious, aware patient, the deliberate decision by the individual to stop dialysis would not be acceptable unless death was imminent from some condition other then renal failure. Suffering should be treated as competently as medically feasible but voluntary, premature death to escape suffering is impermissible.

II. Judaism

There is a wide range in ethical positions from the reform to that of classical orthodox Judaism. The latter is clear in its basic message although individual viewpoints vary. Because of man's unique relationship to, and creation by the Divine, life has special significance, both quantitatively and qualitatively. Suicide is forbidden and every effort has to be made to promote health and longevity. Even the addition of a short time period to the dying person is considered valuable unless suffering is of such magnitude that it eclipses any benefit. To promote health, save life or relieve suffering, numerous religious observations may be disregarded in favour of the greater good. The ill or dying person is obligated to receive treatment and every effort must be taken by the afflicted as well as those caring for him or her, to either restore the person to health or ameliorate their suffering. This singleminded, dedicated, even stringent approach to those who are sick, predicates that treatment cannot and must not be discontinued unless it is clearly futile [8, 9]. Where dialysis or other forms of life support are merely prolonging the dying process, where recovery, even if limited, is impossible then there is agreement that these forms of treatment should be stopped, thereby allowing the termination of life to occur 'naturally' [10]. The sense that only the Creator has the right to decide when this time has arrived is given in this passage from the Siddur.

> My God, the soul which you have placed within me is pure. You have created it; you have fashioned it; you have breathed it into me and you preserve it within me, and you will, at some time, take it from me and return it to me in the time to come [11].

This view of Jewish law or Halakhah, therefore conflicts with the modern ethical stance inherent in the individual's right to self determination and autonomy provided this does not conflict with societal rights. Halakhah, for the Orthodox, has a treasure trove of guidance for today's problems of ethical decision making [12]. The historical precedents and writings related to them, all based ultimately on the Torah, must not be disregarded. While at first no parallel or precedent may be seen, on closer scrutiny by those with the wisdom to understand, a way that is righteous and just will be found.

The principle whereby the individual has the right to forego life sustaining treatment represents an important distinction between Judaic and secular bioethics. As Shimon Glick has expressed it,

> beneficence takes precedence over autonomy [13].

In practical terms, there is the inherent uncertainty, in individual cases, as to whether the person has passed beyond the point of being helped by active treatment. In Halakhah, cessation of respiration signified death [14] but that was prior to the use of endotracheal tubes and respirators. In the setting of the intensive care unit, the absence of respiration calls for mechanical ventilation rather than pronouncement of death. As a result, treatment will be continued unless the medical view is that imminent (within a few days) death is inevitable and that treatment cannot influence this outcome. In most instances in practice, dialysis and other forms of life support are carried on until total collapse of bodily function takes place with the patient's demise a few minutes or hours later.

Movement from this traditional, orthodox viewpoint towards a looser, more liberal Judaism allows a greater range of options and less consistency [15]. Certainly, the importance and primacy attached to human life remains unchanged but there will be found a greater range of individual opinions which are acceptable to the community at large. The views of reform Judaism as they concern life support would overlap those of secular humanists. Mechanical and intrusive methods would be discarded once the chances of any recovery became increasingly unlikely, allowing death to occur, subsequent to this cessation, from whatever underlying physio-pathological processes are present. A viewpoint that humankind can, to some extent, control their own destinies and that the application of technology serving only to prolong existence is not consonant with man's unique sentient being and hence, its cessation should not cause disquiet. Censure, overt or implicit, by the religious authorities would not follow such a course, whereas, in both the conservative traditions of Islam and Orthodox Judaism such 'premature' hastening of death would be seen as a violation of the Divine prerogative which alone decides the beginning and end of man's time on earth and where an extra second of time may be worth as much or more than years of existence [16].

III. Christianity

For the most part, the major groupings within Christianity would have affinity toward the views discussed previously of reform Judaism and secular humanism as they apply to life support. In fact, one of the most renowned Protestant ethicists of this century. Reinhold Niebuhr has argued the impossibility of deriving a social ethic (read biomedical ethic) from a pure religious ethic ...

> (it) is not applicable to the problems of contemporary society nor yet to any conceivable society [17].

The uncertainty, the sense of continuing to understand and learn as we go along is very much a feature of Christian Protestant and, to an increasing extent, Roman Catholic biomedical ethics. This is expressed by Paul Ramsey in his influential writing 'The Patient as Person' when he states that

> Medical ethics today must, indeed, be 'casuistry'; .... we can no longer be so confident that 'resolution' or 'solution' will be forthcoming [18].

The source for these views lies in epistemology. In particular, the importance placed on the foundation writings, the New Testament and, to a lesser extent, the Old Testament or Hebrew Bible. Unlike the Quran, which is considered to be as authoritative today as it was when written by the Prophet and to

> represent the ultimate and permanent source of guidance [19].

the New Testament is viewed differently by most biblical scholars [20]. The writings are not verbatim accounts of what Jesus said but rather they acquired their present form over many years with considerable selection and filtering in order to serve an expository function for whichever group the author was writing. The words of Jesus which have come down to us are applied to present day ethics only with varying degrees of license. The principles however; love, consideration, justice, concern, equality, dignity, stewardship and so on, remain valid. They have shaped the teaching of some of the most influential ethicists of our time [21]. These attributes are now universally accepted, in theory at least if not always in practice; however, their applications in individual cases may be problematic because of conflicting claims and rights.

It should be noted that within most Christian sub-groups, there are those who read the New Testament literally and would apply whatever is found there to problems of today with little, if any, further modification or adjustment [20]. To them the Bible is the Word of God and therefore revered and followed in the same way as the Quran is for Islam. Ethical conduct for contraception, abortion, sexuality, marriage and so on, would then be dependent on biblical exegesis.

A. *Roman Catholicism*

The official teaching of the Church, as it concerns life-sustaining treatment and its use or non-use, is perhaps best expressed in a position statement from the Vatican in 1980 [22]. The current position has not changed. Life is seen as a gift of God with the use of that gift to be enjoyed in the service and love of God. Thus, the taking of life is prohibited, whether by 'mercy killing', suicide, abortion, or homicide. Suffering is seen as an inescapable aspect of our humanity. The use of technology to mitigate and relieve suffering is acceptable, even if to do so may indirectly shorten life. Here the intention is not to produce death but to give relief. Artificial methods of life support are permissible, indeed encouraged, but are not always mandatory and may be discarded if their use becomes unhelpful or if suffering is unrelieved and unremitting, or when the burden of treatment is disproportionate to any benefit that may ensue.

The contrast between this view and the views of Orthodox Judaism and Islam is striking [23]. Its origin lies in the Jesus of the New Testament who voluntarily followed a path to early death entailing much suffering but who overcame death to be with his Father. Thus, the Roman Catholic Church sees suffering and death as something to be avoided but, if unavoidable, then potentially the faithful may share in Christ's sufferings [24]. Death, in itself, is not the end and therefore its inevitability does not have to be circumvented at all costs because beyond death lies paradise. The confluence of the Western democratic ideal –

over himself. . . . the individual is sovereign [25]

with the ecclesiastical view that:

The time may come, therefore, when someone is reasonably convinced that life is coming to an end, and a prolongation of dying by additional complicated medical treatment is not the best investment the person can make of what remains [26].

highlights the importance of autonomy and self-determination in the dying process, once it has progressed to a certain stage.

While the Catholic is willing to make use of modern technology, this is not always mandatory and there are no difficulties in abandoning treatment which fails to meet expectations. Cure is not to be pursued at all costs because there is a more fundamental good which, if not attained in this life, will await the believer in the next.

B. *Protestantism*

We are faced here with literally hundreds of different groupings, each with their own interpretation of the 'truth' as they see it. However, the mainline churches, Lutheran, Methodist, Anglican (Episcopal), and United hold views very similar to those of Roman Catholicism when it concerns the termination of life support. The majority are strongly opposed to deliberate abbreviation of life as distinct from discontinuing treatment that is futile or merely prolonging the dying process. This is well expressed in the following excerpts;

> Christians know that death is not just an end but an opening to eternal life. Because we human beings have an eternal destiny, individuals have no right, even in the name of altruism, to cut short the earthly preparation of innocent human beings.

> To prolong dying is not a doctor's duty . . .

> Life supporting equipment such as respirators or dialysis machines, [should not] be withdrawn from patients who are not dying and who need them . . . This is not to be confused with the removal of a machine from a dying patient whose condition cannot be improved by it' [27].

IV. The significance of religious beliefs

The foregoing has looked briefly at a normative position of each of the three major world religions. It may be asked: To what extent do the faithful, in practice, actually follow and abide by these precepts?

There is little, if any, data on this subject in relation to life support. In a discussion on 'Exclusion from dialysis' in 1981, Fox at no point discusses religious constraints although the analysis focuses on sociological rather than medical and technical aspects [28]. There are at least six publications dealing with withdrawal of dialysis. They originate from Canada [29, 30], the United States [31, 32], and Sweden [33, 34]. In none of these are religious factors mentioned by the authors. In a series of letters to the New England Journal of Medicine, in response to the Minneapolis paper, none of the correspondents refer to religion as a factor either for or against discontinuing treatment [35] and it is also not considered in an ethical forum on dialysis withdrawal [36]. The reasons for this could be varied. The most obvious is that, faced with such an overwhelming, life threatening event as terminating dialysis, religious beliefs become unimportant. We would question this interpretation. All these studies have been retrospective and none have examined specifically the importance of religious values in the decision-making. As society is largely secular (although many nominally adhere to some religious group), the import of belief would be largely diluted. A recent prospective survey of hospitalized patients sought their attitude towards life support and the conditions determining refusal of such therapy [37]. Again, religion was not discussed, suggesting either its lack of importance or possibly that religious views cannot be quantified. Perhaps they are too indefinite or that their consideration may actually be 'unscientific' and unfitting for a dispassionate, learned study!

Against these views is a remarkable paper showing that deaths of Jews were fewer than expected prior to the Passover in Los Angeles and higher after the holiday [38]. This pattern was not present in Blacks, Orientals and Jewish infants. The indication is that death was in some way delayed to permit celebration of the religious event. We would interpret this as suggesting that religiosity is indeed very important but readily overlooked unless specifically looked for or studied in a homogeneous group of religious adherents. Thus, the 'official' statements by leading figures of the various religious groupings may well reflect, to some degree, the views of the 'people in the street' who are silent worshippers in the shrine, synagogue or church of their choice. If such indeed is the case, then care-giving professionals need to know more about the religious convictions of those they are trying to help. It would also be desirable for them to have at least a rudimentary understanding of some of the world's religions. Such an understanding could itself be beneficial in a world that is segmented and divided into multiple component parts. These divisions engender distrust and prejudice rather than tolerance and understanding. Patients' attitudes and coping mechanisms, in response to present day technology, will be influenced, not solely by their social and family ties, but also for many, by religious views and beliefs that originated millenia previously. Moving from Islam through Judaism, to Christianity the weight and significance of these views for the individual, and the society in which they live, become progressively diluted and secularized. However, their importance cannot be trivialized and we believe this to be particularly relevant for care-givers working in areas of life support.

V. Refusal of treatment

Differences of opinion may occur when patients wish to stop dialysis and their physicians believe they should continue. Frequently the wish to stop arises from a variety of social and/or medical concerns which are amenable to alteration. Given the appropriate modifications, these individuals may be content to continue treat-

124

ment and some might eventually be transplanted. There are a few however, in whom further improvement is apparently impossible, yet the physician's reluctance to stop treatment is at odds with the patient's wish to do so. The patients may have carefully considered the significance of their wishes as it affects their relationship with God and decided on this course, whereas the physician remains committed to a technological alternative. This dilemma is a particularly North American one and its resolution lies in the right of the individual to decide whether he or she does, or does not, want treatment. This is acknowledged for the competent individual, provided the person understands the significance and complications of stopping treatment. The rare instances where this right has been overridden has been described previously [39]. These exceptions indicate the general rule that the competent individual, has the choice to either consent to, or refuse even life saving treatment for their own (religious or other) reasons.

Acknowledgements

I would like to thank Rev. Dr. L. James, Rev. D. W. Stinebrickner and Drs. A.A.N. Al Shimemeri and M. Vasilevsky for their helpful suggestions and manuscript review, my wife, Margot, for her assistance and Ms. J. Sears for secretarial help.

References

1. Quran. The meaning of the Glorious Koran. Mentor. 2;30.
2. Sahin AF. Islamic Transplantation Ethics. Transpl Proc 1990; 22: (3): 939.
3. Quran 39: 42.
4. Darsh SM. Islamic health rules. Abul Qasim Publications, Jeddah, Saudi Arabia.
5. Hathout H. Islamic basis for biomedical ethics. Fidia Research Foundation Symposium, Transcultural dimensions of medical ethics. National Academy of Sciences, Washington, D.C. April 26–27 1990.
6. Darsh SM. ibid.
7. Quran 40: 67, 68.
8. Riemer J, (ed). Jewish Reflections on Death 1974; Schocken Books: New York.
9. Glick S. A view from Sinai – A Jewish perspective on biomedical ethics. Fidia Symposium, ibid.
10. Life-sustaining treatment: New York State task force on life and the law. July, 1987.
11. Rosner F, Bleich JD (eds). Quoted by Bleich JD in Jewish Bioethics. Sanhedrin Press: New York 1979: p. 292.
12. ibid.
13. Glick S, ibid.
14. Solovachik A. The Halakhic definition of death. In Jewish bioethics. ibid.
15. Life sustaining treatment. ibid.
16. See Comments by Bleich JD in Jewish Bioethics. The Quinlan case: A Jewish perspective. ibid.
17. Niebuhr R. An interpretation of Christian ethics. Seaburg Press, New York 1979; p. 31.
18. Ramsey P. The patient as person. Yale University Press 1970; p. 17.
19. Bucaille M. The Qur'an and modern science. Abul Qasim Publications: Jeddah, Saudi Arabia.
20. Kee HC, Young FW, Froehlich K. Understanding the New Testament. 3rd Edn. Prentice-Hall, Inc 1973.

21. See: J Med and Philosophy 1990; 15 (3).
22. Declaration on Euthanasia, the Sacred Congregation for the Doctrine of the Faith. Vatican City, 1980. In: Deciding to forego life-sustaining treatment. President's Commission for the Study of Ethical Problems in Medicine and Biomedical and Behavioural Research. U.S. Government Printing Office 1983.
23. See: Life Support – Religious Considerations 1987 In Proc. 2nd international congress on ethics in medicine. New York.
24. Philipp 3: 10. Common Bible. Revised Standard Version, Collins, 1972, p. 186.
25. Mill JS. On Liberty. Penguin Books 1984; p. 69.
26. Ashley BM, O'Rourke KD. Health care ethics. A theological analysis. The Catholic Health Association of the United States 1982; p. 38.
27. Grant S, Gentles I (ed): Euthanasia in care for the dying and bereaved. Anglican Book Center 1982.
28. Fox RC. Exclusion from dialysis: A sociological and legal perspective. Kidney Int 1981; 19: 739–751.
29. Rodin GM, Chmara BA, Ennis J et al. Stopping life-sustaining medical treatment: Psychiatric considerations in the termination of renal dialysis. Can J Psychiatry 1981; 26: 540–4.
30. Hirsch DJ. Death from dialysis termination. Nephrol Dial Transplant 1989; 4: 41–4.
31. McKegney FP, Lange P. The decision to no longer live on chronic hemodialysis. Amer J Psychiat 1971; 128: (3): 47–54.
32. Neu S, Kjellstrand CM. Stopping long-term dialysis: an empirical study of withdrawal of life-supporting treatment. New Engl J Med 1986; 314: 14–20.
33. Silva JEM, Kjellstrand CM. Withdrawing life support. Do families and physicians decide as patients do? Nephron 1988; 48: 201–205.
34. Roberts JC, Kjellstrand CM. Choosing death. Withdrawal from chronic dialysis without medical reason. Acta Med Scand 1988; 223: 181–6.
35. Dessner GH, Fisher SH, Curry E et al. Stopping long-term dialysis. New Engl J Med 1986; 314 (22): 1449–51.
36. Lowance DC, Singer PA, Siegler M. Withdrawal from dialysis: an ethical perspective. Kidney Int 1988; 34: 124–35.
37. Frankl D, Oye RK, Bellamy PE. Attitudes of hospitalized patients toward life support: A survey of 200 medical inpatients. Amer J Med 1989; 86: 645–8.
38. Phillips DP, King EW. Death takes a holiday: Mortality surrounding major social occasions. Lancet 1988; 2: 728–729.
39. Kaye M, Bourgouin P, Low G. Physician's non-compliance with patients' refusal of life-sustaining treatment. Amer J Nephrol 1987; 7: 304–312.

10. Legal aspects of stopping dialysis

RONALD CRANFORD

This chapter will explore three major questions: in general, what is the current state of the law on termination of treatment decisions as we begin the 1990s, what is the current law on stopping treatment in dialysis patients, and what are the unique features of stopping dialysis that make these decisions more, or less, legally problematic?

I. Current law

Legal and ethical dilemmas surrounding decisions to stop treatment are of relatively recent vintage. Legal decisions concerning the stopping of any form of medical treatment were essentially unheard of before the mid-1970s; emergence of the legal aspects of termination of treatment decisions can be traced to the *Quinlan* decision in 1975–76 before the trial court and then the State Supreme Court of New Jersey. Since, then, the number of cases before the courts have increased almost exponentially. In *The Right to Die*, Alan Meisel cites 59 'significant reported' right-to-die legal cases in the United States from 1975 to 1990 [1]. With regard to the withdrawal of artificial nutrition and hydration from critically ill patients, no significant cases came before the courts prior to 1983. During the period 1983 to the present, however, at least 50 court cases have focused on the withdrawal of this specific form of treatment [2]. According to a report from the National Center of State Courts, there have been at least 7,000 court cases on termination of treatment in the United States [3].

In addition to court cases, there also has been a great deal of activity in the state legislatures [4, 5]. Most states now have some form of advance directive legislation, e.g., living wills (41 states and the District of Columbia), or durable powers of attorney for health care (29 states and the District of Columbia). The courts and the legislatures have been somewhat divergent in their views, however. The courts, through a series of decisions, have tended to expand the rights of individual patients to discontinue treatment while the legislatures have in some ways restricted those same rights. Many living will statutes limit the termination of treatment to only those patients who are 'terminally ill'. Until recently, legislation in six states

127

(Missouri, Connecticut, Wisconsin, Oklahoma, Maine, Georgia) forbids the withdrawal of artificial nutrition and hydration under nearly all circumstances [6]. The Child and Abuse Amendment of 1984 also narrowly defines the circumstances in which nutrition and hydration may be stopped on critically ill newborns, though the language is unclear and the intent confusing [7].

Gradually, though, over the last fifteen years the legal system (in case law or statutes) has increasingly recognized the common law right of competent patients to refuse treatment. In 1990, the U.S. Supreme Court in *Cruzan* recognized a federal constitutional right of patients to forgo medical treatment. Some state courts have also recognized that patients have a state constitutional right to stop treatment.

A consensus is beginning to develop on some of the issues surrounding termination of treatment. A consensus is emerging, for example, that not only do competent patients have a constitutional and common-law right to discontinue treatment, but also that incompetent patients share in this same legal right. Further, a consensus is developing that not only respirators, but all forms of medical treatment may be discontinued.

However, at least two major issues remain legally problematic. The first issue concerns incompetent patients: what procedural mechanisms should be established to protect their rights, and who is the appropriate surrogate decision-maker? [8] Some states have now erected stringent procedural safeguards for withdrawing treatment from incompetent patients. The New Jersey Supreme Court, acting partly from a lack of faith in the medical profession, recommended in the *Conroy* decision a complicated system for protecting the rights of incompetent patients [9]. However, this system, which included the involvement of the State Ombudsman's Office, turned out to be completely unworkable [10].

A second major issue that remains controversial is the withdrawal of artificial nutrition and hydration; however, here too a consensus seems to be emerging. All appellate court decisions (except for *Cruzan* in Missouri and *Grant* in Washington) have concluded that medical means of providing artificial nutrition and hydration are comparable to other life-sustaining medical treatments and can be discontinued according to the same principles and practices followed in the withdrawal of other forms of treatment [9, 11–19]. Medical organizations and interdisciplinary authorities have articulated the same view [20–23]. However, there continues to be some conflict between the parties moving toward consensus (i.e., medical organizations, interdisciplinary authorities and the courts) and other deliberative bodies, such as some state legislatures and perhaps federal lawmakers.

Besides addressing the substantive questions of what constitutes medical treatment, and which medical conditions (terminally ill, imminently dying, permanently comatose, hopelessly ill) are appropriate for termination of treatment, the courts have tried to determine the best way to resolve who should make decisions for incompetents and how those decisions should be made [24]. 'Substituted judgment' and 'best interests' are two common legal concepts. According to the standard of substituted judgment (which is considered subjective and highly individualistic), the decision to withdraw treatment is made after considering what the patient would have wanted. The more evidence there is of the patient's likely wishes (previous oral statements, written statements, and general life style), the more the standard of substituted judgment is satisfied. This standard does not specify who should decide, only that the surrogate decisionmaker act in accordance with the patient's wishes. The 'best interests' standard is used when it is not known what the patient would have wanted. There is a great deal of confusion in both the legal and ethical literature on what constitutes 'best interests'. This standard is often followed by weighing the benefits and burdens of treatment against the benefits and burdens of continued existence for the patient.

Some states have adopted a more stringent evidentiary standard than others with regard to substituted judgment and have developed elaborate procedural standards to minimize abuse. That is, some states require more evidence than do other states as to the patient's likely wishes before they will accept that the substituted judgment standard has been satisfied. Most recently, State Supreme Court decisions in three states (Missouri, Maine, and New York) have articulated 'clear and convincing evidence' standards [17, 25–28]. Exactly how to apply these standards is a different matter. Individual trial court judges are free to decide whether the patient's previous views and life style meet a clear and convincing evidence standard. This standard then is highly individualistic, varying according to the particular trial court judge applying it. Other states have been less stringent in developing an evidentiary standard for incompetent patients. For example, the Minnesota State Supreme Court in *Torres* had little evidence of what Mr. Torres would have wanted, and seemed to lean more toward a best interests standard [29].

Some states seem to place greater confidence in the family or friends to make decisions for incompetents, while other states have been reluctant to entrust family and health care providers with these decisions.

With this variety of judicial approaches to the termination of treatment, it should be remembered that in this country, decisions to limit treatment are made thousands of times each day – often in circumstances where the evidence of what the patient wants falls well short of a clear and convincing evidence standard, where the diagnosis and prognosis are less certain than the diagnosis of the persistent vegetative state, and where there is less unanimity among the immediate family members concerning the appropriate action. Recent studies have indicated that there may be at least one million deaths each year in the United States in which a conscious decision is made to limit treatment in some way [30]. Very few of these cases reach the courts, nor could the courts, by whatever procedural mechanism they recommend, ever rule on even 1 % of these cases in a strictly judicial setting.

What happens, then, when a ruling such as the *Saikewicz* decision by the Supreme Judicial Court in Massachusetts appears to require routine judicial review for all cases involving incompetent patients? [31, 32]. In reality, what occurs is that these cases are not reviewed by the courts, and often treatment is continued far beyond the time when it should be discontinued (because of the fear of legal repercussions), or, the appropriate decisions are made, but more surreptitiously and quietly than they should be. Ultraconservative decisions advocating some form of routine judicial review in most termination of treatment decisions in incompetent patients will never work. There needs to be some compromise wherein the courts articulate policy, in conjunction with the legislatures, while ensuring their ability to resolve the more legally problematic cases. Since we are still basically in our infancy regarding the legal aspects of termination of treatment, how this area unfolds is still uncertain and will vary significantly in the individual states.

How does all of this relate to dialysis? What are the unique features of stopping dialysis that make this practice more or less legally problematic. Finally, how much have the courts been involved in dialysis cases?

II. Court cases

Of the major cases before the courts in this country on stopping treatment, only two have directly involved dialysis as the primary treatment to be discontinued. Earle N. Spring, 77, suffered from severe dementia ('advanced senility') and end-stage renal disease [33], and received 5-hour hemodialysis treatments three times a week. Heavy sedation was often used to overcome his resistance to treatment, and he often resisted transportation to dialysis treatment and pulled the dialysis needles out of his arm. Mr. Spring experienced leg cramps, headaches, and dizziness as side effects of the dialysis.

In January, 1979, his wife of 55 years and his only son petitioned the probate court in Massachusetts for an order directing that dialysis be discontinued. The son had been appointed temporary guardian of his father, but in view of the request to discontinue treatment, the probate court also appointed a guardian *ad litem* to represent Mr. Spring.

The probate court judge ruled in favour of discontinuing treatment but this decision was appealed by the guardian *ad litem* in December 1979 – almost one year after the court proceedings had begun. When the intermediate appellate court in Massachusetts affirmed the probate court's decision, the guardian *ad litem* appealed again. After 15 months of hearings, appeals, reversals, and stays the Massachusetts Supreme Judicial Court (SJC) finally issued its decision, one month after Mr. Spring had died.

A major reason why the Massachusetts SJC decided to hear Mr. Spring's case is that this case gave the court an opportunity to clarify what it had said in a previous decision in the matter of Joseph Saikewicz [34]. In *Saikewicz*, the Massachusetts SJC appeared to say that all cases involving the discontinuation of treatment in incompetent patients should be a matter of routine judicial involvement [35, 45]. In *Spring*, the court took the opportunity to say that this was not the intent of the *Saikewicz* decision. The justices clearly indicated that judicial approval was not always required before stopping treatment on incompetent patients. The court identified the following issues to be considered: the extent of impairment of the patient's mental faculties; whether the patient is in the custody of a state institution; the prognosis with or without proposed treatment; the complexity, risk, and novelty of such treatment; its possible side effects; the patient's level of understanding and probable reaction; the urgency of the decision; the consent of the patient's spouse or guardian; the good faith of those who participate in the decision; the clarity of professional opinion as to good medical practice; the interests of third persons; and the administrative requirements of any institution involved [36].

Unfortunately, the court did not prioritize these issues, nor did it indicate which ones needed to be reviewed by the probate courts in Massachusetts. Regarding criminal or civil liability for physicians in termination of treatment decisions, the Massachusetts SJC said, 'Little need be said about criminal liability: there is precious 'little precedent and what there is suggests that the doctor will be protected if he acts on a good faith judgment that is not grievously unreasonable by medical standards' [36].

Another case involving dialysis occurred in the State of New York in 1982 [37]. Peter Cinque, a 41-year-old diabetic, was blind, had partial amputations of both legs, a bleeding gastrointestinal ulcer, and cardiovascular disease – all due to complications of diabetes. In addition to these complications, Mr. Cinque was undergoing dialysis several days a week for end-stage renal disease. He was said to be receiving analgesic medications, including Demerol, for great pain, but was described as mentally alert and competent.

In early October, 1982, because of the pain and other complications Mr. Cinque decided that he wished to discontinue dialysis and be allowed to die at home in the presence of his family. This decision was discussed with the entire family and a Catholic priest. Mr. Cinque had several conversations with his nephrologist on October 12 and 14. The nephrologist and administrators at Lydia Hall Hospital told Mr. Cinque he could stop his dialysis on October 15. Before this termination of treatment, he was removed from all sedative and analgestic medication so that he could be examined by two psychiatrists to determine his competency and ability to make his own decisions. After these examinations, he was found 'coherent and relevant' and unequivocal in his desire to stop dialysis and be allowed to die. On the same day he was examined, Mr. Cinque signed two documents expressing his wishes (since he was blind, he signed with a mark).

Mark Cinque, one of Mr. Cinque's brothers, commented that Peter Cinque 'was at last comforted and relieved' when the hospital appeared to agree with his wishes to discontinue dialysis. However, several hours later, the hospital had not only refused to discontinue treatment, but had gone to court. Mark Cinque described his brother as going through 'the most painful period of agony and suffering I had ever seen'[38].

Two days later, Mr. Cinque sustained a respiratory arrest after which he lapsed into a coma and was maintained on a respirator. A trial court judge visited the bedside on October 19 and 21, 1982 and found him to be unconscious both times.

The guardian *ad litem* appointed by the court agreed with the family that Mr. Cinque had left unequivocal expressions of what he wanted prior to his present comatose state. The lower court found in favor of stopping treatment, but the case was immediately appealed to the highest court in New York, the Court of Appeals. The New York high court took the opportunity of Mr. Cinque's dilemma to clarify its previous decisions in *Eichner* and *Storar* [25, 39] in which a clear and convincing evidence standard of the patient's wishes had been established before treatment could be stopped. The trial court judge felt that Mr. Cinque's expressions before losing consciousness were so compelling that his statements satisfied a much more stringent standard than even 'clear and convincing,' that of 'beyond a reasonable doubt' and ordered the hospital to discontinue treatment on October 22. Unfortunately, in a bizarre and cruel turn of events, the hospital discontinued treatment immediately upon hearing of the court's decision without allowing his family to be present at Mr. Cinque's bedside. Commenting on the Cinque case, Willard Gaylin, President of the Hastings Center, asked: 'How did we get into this 'Alice-in-Wonderland' world, where a man must beg for his legal rights, prove his sanity, endure court hearings, and finally be reduced to a living cadaver to do what has generally been accepted as his privilege?' [40]

It is ironic that the day before Mr. Cinque finally was allowed to die, the President's Commission for the Study of Ethical Problems in Medicine released a report on informed consent, pointing out that 4 of 5 Americans believe that the processes by which patients grant prior consent for hospital treatment are merely 'legal maneuvers to protect doctors from lawsuits' [41]. The commission's Chairman, Morris B. Abrams, an attorney in New York City, called this finding 'dismal and startling' [41]. The commission said that in order for informed consent to be an effective process, it must be part of a larger process of shared decision making and mutual respect between physician and patient. No case could more dramatically illustrate the failure of 'informed consent', 'shared decision-making,' and 'mutual respect between physician and patient' than the clash between Peter Cinque and medical and administrative personnel at Lydia Hall Hospital.

What general observations can we make from the Spring and Cinque cases, and how they were handled by the courts? First, quality of life was a major issue in both cases. It was obvious that quality of life was poor for both Mr. Spring and Mr. Cinque. Both situations are typical scenarios in which dialysis is often discontinued. In a study done by Neu and Kjellstrand of 66 patients who were incompetent at the time of stopping dialysis, 37 (56%) had 'advanced arteriosclerotic or dialysis dementia' and another 6 (9%) had severe memory/intellectual deficits that were secondary to strokes [42]. In many of these cases, dialysis was stopped for the same reasons it was discontinued in Mr. Spring.

Second, the courts seemed to view dialysis as a medical treatment with clear-cut benefits and side effects, and treated the termination of dialysis like the termination of other forms of medical treatment. The courts viewed stopping dialysis as being much less controversial than stopping artificial nutrition and hydration, or stopping life-saving medical treatment such as blood transfusions.

Third, these two cases reflect the early days of legal analysis. *Spring* was one of the earliest cases to reach the appellate court level in the United States (after *Quinlan, Saikewicz,* and *Dinnerstein*) [31, 43, 44]. In Massachusetts, the higher courts were trying to clarify what they had said in *Saikewicz*, the second major right-to-die case in this country.

Fourth, the Cinque case illustrates how much easier it is for the courts to resolve issues when the patient is competent and his or her wishes concerning quality of life and medical treatment are clearly known. It also supports the movement towards advance directives. Thus, the courts focused on issues involving competent patients and the legal principle of substituted judgment rather than best interests. In the *Spring* case, however, the legal analysis focused more on the best interests standard. There was little offered at the probate-court level to identify what Mr. Spring would have wanted, other than his wife's assertion, based on their long years of marriage, that 'he wouldn't want to live.' The higher court also took note of the fact that Mr. Spring had led a vigorous active life, which he was no longer able to do.

Finally, Peter Cinque's dilemma exemplifies the extraordinary concerns about the liability of hospital and medical personnel. This concern about potential criminal and civil liability borders on hysteria; as in Mr. Cinque's case, it compromises the ability of the medical profession to act in a humane, compassionate, common-sense way and brutalizes the patient and his family. It is hard to justify the actions of the hospital and physicians in his case, but three factors may partially explain what transpired. First, the case occurred at a time in the right-to-die movement when the law was much more unsettled than it is today. Second, the case was litigated in the State of New York, where the preoccupation with liability to the detriment of common sense and humane care is as great as it is anywhere in the country. Third, the highest court in New York had recently established an extremely high standard for knowing what incompetent patients would have wanted (erecting the clear and convincing evidence standard in the matters of *Eichner* and *Storar*); and physicians and hospital administrators may have been unclear on the full ramifications of these legal decisions.

Three other legal cases involving dialysis should be mentioned. In 1979, the Massachusetts SJC affirmed a trial-court order compelling an unconsenting, competent adult prisoner to submit to dialysis treatments that were considered life-saving [46]. The higher court found that the prisoner's right to refuse life-saving treatment was outweighed by the state's interests in preserving life, in maintaining the ethical integrity of the medical profession and permitting hospitals to fully care for their patients, and in upholding orderly prison administration. This ruling, however, should not be considered a major legal decision on dialysis because it involved unique features of a termination of treatment decision not often seen. Essentially, the court felt that the prisoner was seeking to circumvent restrictions of the prison system by refusing dialysis.

A Minnesota case will help to dispel two commonly held myths in right-to-die cases, myths that have no solid foundation in theory or practice. The first is that there is a real possibility of civil or criminal liability in situations where the cases have been handled well by health care providers. The second myth, closely related to the first, is that family members, near or distant, who were not involved in the decision-making process leading to termination of treatment, may come forward at some later date and successfully sue physicians, even when the cases were handled well. A major problem, one that further perpetuates these fallacious views, is that many physicians seem to want complete immunity from civil or criminal liability for their actions, no matter how well or poorly they handle individual cases. To these physicians, any risk is too much risk. Their concerns about doing good for the individual patient are far outweighed by their concerns about liability. If individual cases are not handled well, either procedurally or substantively, then physicians should run a risk of sanction in some form, e.g., when a physician does not make a good faith effort to find family or friends or other appropriate surrogate decision makers for an incompetent patient, or when a physician does not fully inform the patient of all the relevant benefits and risks of alternative forms of therapy. But, when the physicians handle cases appropriately, then the real risk of liability is small.

During the early 1970s a 62-year-old woman on chronic peritoneal dialysis in a large midwestern dialysis program became progressively demented and unable to care for herself at home. In the hospital, she would scream for no apparent reason, and her behavior became increasingly disturbing to other patients. After numerous discussions with her husband which were extensively documented in the medical records, the attending nephrologist, with the consent of the husband, decided to discontinue dialysis, and the patient died shortly thereafter. Six months later, the patient's husband died.

Three years after the patient's death, shortly before the statute of limitations would have expired, two of the patient's children filed a civil law suit for abandonment against the nephrologist and the hospital. The plaintiffs argued that the nephrologist had abandoned the patient simply because he had discontinued dialysis. The decision was divided into two parts. First, the jury found that the defendants were not liable. The nephrologist had done nothing wrong legally by stopping dialysis on this patient with an extremely poor prognosis. Second, the jury found there would have been no monetary damages awarded to the plaintiffs, even if the physician had been found guilty of malpractice. Since the patient was totally disabled because of her illness, the jury reasoned no financial loss could result from her death.

Afterwards, one member of the jury asked the physician, 'Why did it take so long to make the decision (to discontinue dialysis)?' [47] Hopefully, this case will contribute to the view that doctors, acting in good faith and in accordance with reasonable standards of medical practice, need not fear frivolous law suits brought by disgruntled relatives.

Another court case involving dialysis occurred in New Mexico in 1983. The legal guardian for James R. Smith petitioned the lower court to authorize discontinuation of hemodialysis. This request was granted. However, the lower court's ruling was reversed on appeal to the Supreme Court of New Mexico who stated that there was no statute in New Mexico that would empower a guardian to discontinue hemodialysis on behalf of an incompetent patient. After this unfortunate ruling, the New Mexico legislature amended the state's right-to-die act by providing that, when an incompetent patient not executing a document under the right-to-die act is certified as terminally ill or in an irreversible coma, the physician may be allowed to remove medical treatment when all family members agree in good faith that the patient, if competent, would have chosen to forgo treatment. Thus, this case served as a stimulus for the New Mexico legislature to expand the rights of surrogates to discontinue treatment, and, indirectly, to expand the rights of patients to allow decisions to be made for them after they become incompetent [48].

III. Unique features of dialysis

What are the unique features of the withdrawal of dialysis that distinguishes it from the withdrawal of other forms of medical treatment? Why have there been so few dialysis cases before the courts? Will this trend of minimal legal involvement continue? What are the characteristics of cases involving cessation of dialysis that seem to make these decisions less legally troublesome?

A. *Dialysis as 'high-tech' medical treatment*

Where does dialysis lie on the continuum from highly technological, complicated, expensive, and burdensome medical treatments (e.g., respirators, cardiopulmonary resuscitation, heart-lung machines, extracorporeal membrane oxygenators) to simpler, less technological, less expensive and relatively nonburdensome medical treatments (e.g., antibiotics, artificial nutrition and hydration)? It seems clear that dialysis is perceived to be closer to the complex, technologic end of the continuum, thus decisions to stop dialysis are less legally problematic than decisions to forgo forms of treatment at the more basic end of the continuum.

Another reason why stopping dialysis may be less legally controversial is that in some cases it provides a stop-gap measure until transplantation can be done. When transplantation cannot be performed, or one or more transplants are unsuccessful, dialysis is still a treatment that is unquestionably life-prolonging. However, there often comes a time during the course of the progressive disease and its medical complications when the side effects of dialysis (which are rarely inconsequential, even in the early stages of renal failure) exceed the benefits. The long-term use of dialysis and subsequent determinations that its effectiveness has run its course and that it is now no longer beneficial, satisfies the medical-ethical (and legal) standard of a 'time-limited trial' of therapy [21].

B. *Competent patients*

Decisions to stop dialysis are often made by competent patients who have experienced the benefits and burdens of dialysis over a relatively long period of time, thus, there is no need to apply a substituted judgment or best interests standard, since the patient makes the decision as a direct expression of autonomy or self-determination. However, while many patients are clearly competent, others are comatose, severely demented, or their competency is unclear. These cases are more legally perplexing.

C. *Quality of life*

Decisions to discontinue dialysis are usually made after the treatment has been given an adequate trial, in order to see how much it helps the patient and to weigh the benefits and burdens of continued treatment in light of the progress of the underlying disease. In the Earle Spring case, for example, the family became convinced that dialysis should be discontinued because Mr. Spring had deteriorated mentally to the point where the family did not think dialysis was prolonging any meaningful existence. Similarly, Peter Cinque decided that the complications of diabetes were so devastating that he no longer wished to continue living with such severe disability and suffering. Hence, some decisions are made after considering the advantages and disadvantages of both dialysis and other forms of treatment. The quality of life in cases resembling Earle Spring and Peter Cinque was so overwhelmingly poor that most people would not dispute decisions to discontinue dialysis. Unlike comparatively simple treatment such as antibiotics or artificial nutrition and hydration, the side effects, expense, and inconvenience of dialysis can be significant – especially when it sustains only marginal quality of life for the patient.

Dialysis is not curative; it does not cure the underlying disease process leading to kidney failure, nor is it life-saving in the same sense that surgery or blood transfusions sometimes are. It sustains life by replacing a basic biological function, as do respirators and artificial nutrition and hydration. Dialysis is an 'artificial kidney,' just as a respirator is an 'artificial lung,' or artificial nutrition and hydration is an 'artificial gastrointestinal system.' Decisions to discontinue dialysis are no different from decisions to discontinue a respirator or to discontinue artificial nutrition and hydration. It is primarily the basic underlying condition of the patient that usually makes the treatment more or less advantageous or detrimental, and not the treatment itself. Decisions to discontinue dialysis, then, are often based not on the change in the benefit or burden accompanying the dialysis treatments themselves, but on the underlying quality of life of the patient. This is especially true when diabetes ravages the body and mind. If a patient has good health in all other respects, there should be little legal controversy surrounding a decision to continue dialysis. The improved quality of life would be such that most patients would accept the side effects of dialysis.

In many respects, then, dialysis decisions are less legally controversial than other non-treatment circumstances. However, three other features may make these cases more legally problematic.

D. *Definition of terminal condition*

The definition of 'terminal condition' has been significantly expanded and modified recently, and this has great bearing on the dialysis issue. In the 1985 version of the Uniform Rights of the Terminally Ill Act (URITA), a terminal condition was defined as a condition in which the patient would die within a relatively short period of time *with* continued medical treatment [49]. According to the newer and much broader definition of terminal condition in the more recent URITA (1989), the patient will die within a relatively short period of time *without* medical treatment [50], thus, any patient who requires continuous life support systems to keep him or her alive and whose medical condition is 'incurable and irreversible' could be considered terminal. A patient in a persistent vegetative state, even though capable of living for an extended period of time (years, or decades) is terminal because he or she would die within a relatively short time (3–30 days, usually 7–14 days) after stopping artificial hydration. Recent court decisions (*Greenspan* in Illinois) have begun to reflect this newer definition [51]. Renal failure by itself, as long as it is incurable and irreversible, could be considered a terminal condition; without continued dialysis the patient will die within a relatively short time, usually only a few weeks.

The newer definition of terminal condition gives patients greater control over their own lives. But this also means that the patient may elect to discontinue dialysis for reasons some would find questionable, such as temporary depression, marital strife, or other reasons that are more psychosociologic than medical.

E. *Static versus progressive disease*

In general, it is more legally controversial to discontinue treatment for a static disease process than for a progressive one. For example, withdrawal of the respirator seems to be more legally permissible in cases of a progressive neurologic disease such as amyotrophic lateral sclerosis, but more legally debatable when the patient's neurologic condition is static, as in a cervical cord injury. The courts and others have drawn distinctions between a progressive course and a static course because decisions to discontinue treatment in a static condition could have more negative impact on other categories of patients with a static condition, such as patients with cerebral palsy. This is why the *McAfee* case in Georgia (a man with a cervical cord injury who asked to have his respirator removed) was so controversial, why the disability groups were opposed to letting the courts allow Mr. McAfee make the decision himself [52], and also why the *Bouvia* case in California was so controversial legally [53]. Ms. Bouvia had cerebral palsy her entire life. Her decision to withdraw artificial nutrition and hydration from herself was not, according to some, related to any progressive medical disease or increased suffering, but had more to do with psychological and social reasons.

In that the underlying renal failure is nonprogressive, discontinuation of dialysis could be considered more controversial than discontinuations of other treatment. However, the basic disease process that led to the renal failure and other medical complications may be progressive, as in diabetes, and it is usually the underlying disease process and its effect on the person that is the primary reason for discontinuing dialysis.

F. Cost containment

A legally contentious situation could arise in the future should dialysis not be offered (or be withdrawn) based on social and economic considerations [54]. Such a situation could easily arise as funds for dialysis become more limited than they have been since the enactment of the end-stage renal disease program in 1973. The British seem to encounter little legal difficulty regarding failure to offer dialysis, as opposed to deciding to withdraw it but find it more difficult to stop dialysis than to withhold it. However, the British medical and legal systems are radically different from ours. A lack of litigation in Great Britain may be of little reassurance to those of us in the United States [55], where we seem to have more difficulty stopping treatment than starting it, although as Neu and Kjellstrand's study shows, and as others have now experienced, we have developed a much more humane, rational, common-sense basis for assessing the benefits and burdens of continued treatment and are more willing to discontinue dialysis for justifiable reasons than we have in the past.

IV. Cruzan and constitutional law

What effect does the recent U.S. Supreme Court ruling in the Nancy Cruzan case have on termination of treatment decisions in general, and dialysis decisions in particular? The *Cruzan* case is the first major termination of treatment case to be decided by the U.S. Supreme Court [56]. Its effects could be widespread or narrow, depending upon one's view of the decision [57].

Nancy Cruzan was 25 years old when she was involved in a single-car motor vehicle accident on a rural road in southwest Missouri on January 11, 1983. She was thrown 35 feet from the car and landed face down, causing obstruction of her airway. From the beginning, her prognosis for recovery of cognitive functions was felt to be extremely poor. She evolved into a persistent vegetative state over ensuing months and a gastrostomy tube was placed on February 7, 1983, approximately four weeks after the accident. In 1986, her parents, Joe and Joyce Cruzan, recognized that Nancy was in a persistent vegetative state and that her condition was hopeless. They further realized that Nancy would not want treatment under such circumstances. Nancy was described by her parents and friends as a proud, feisty, independent individual who took great pride in her physical appearance. The Cruzans began learning of similar cases in other states where feeding tubes had been removed from patients in a vegetative state, but they were told by the rehabilitation center where Nancy was staying that the feeding tube could not be removed without a court order.

In 1988, a trial court judge in Missouri ruled that it was permissible to discontinue Nancy's feeding tube in accordance with what the patient would have wanted and what the family wanted [58]. The case was appealed to the Missouri State Supreme Court by the Attorney General of the State of Missouri and by the guardian *ad litem* appointed by the court to represent Nancy's interests. In a radical departure from nine previous appellate court decisions, the Missouri Supreme Court ruled in a 4-to-3 decision that Nancy's feeding tube could not be withdrawn [27]. The family then appealed to the U.S. Supreme Court which affirmed the ruling of the Missouri Supreme Court on June 25, 1990, and decreed that the Missouri courts were permitted (not required) constitutionally to erect a clear and convincing evidence standard for determining what an incompetent patient would have wanted concerning the stopping of artificial feeding.

There undoubtedly will be widespread misunderstanding concerning what the U.S. Supreme Court did and did not say in *Cruzan*, so it is important to understand that the Court's decision was a very narrow one [59] which said in essence, that the states were free to develop procedural safeguards and evidentiary stand-ards they feel appropriate. This is the only direct effect of the Court's ruling in *Cruzan*.

In addition to this narrow finding, however, the Court also made comments (*dicta*) on several other constitutional and legal aspects of stopping treatment which will have some indirect bearing on legal decisions in the individual states. For example, the Court ruled that a competent patient has a federal constitutional right to refuse treatment, but it did not rule on whether this right extends to incompetent patients. Most importantly, the Court, also by way of *dicta*, decided that there was no essential difference between the withdrawal of artificial nutrition and hydration and the withdrawal of other forms of medical treatment.

Further, five of the nine justices, including all of the dissenters, and Justice O'Connor in her concurring opinion, appeared to place great value on advance directives, especially durable power of attorney for health care and other means to designate surrogates for patients who are no longer competent. Justice O'Connor was fairly forceful in her opinion that there may be a constitutional right of liberty for incompetent patients to have treatment stopped when this decision is effectuated by an appropriately determined surrogate decisionmaker. In Justice O'Connor's words, 'I also write separately to emphasize that the Court does not today decide the issue of whether a State must also give effect to the decisions of a surrogate decisionmaker... In my view, such a duty may well be *constitutionally required* to protect the patient's liberty interest in refusing medical treatment' (emphasis added)[56].

V. Conclusion

What conclusions can we draw from this review so that health care providers can be assured that dialysis decisions are correct (both substantively and procedurally) in the eyes of the law? As noted above, dialysis decisions will almost certainly be viewed as less controversial than other termination of treatment decisions such as artificial feeding or blood transfusions. Dialysis is viewed as a medical treatment located toward the technologically complex end of the treatment continuum; the quality of life for patients receiving such treatment is palpably poor. In perhaps half of the cases, the patient is competent and can make decisions consistent with his or her values. In other cases, family members or friends are available to make decisions for the patient, in terms of either what the patient would have wanted (substituted judgment standard), or what the family or friends perceive to be best for their loved one (best interests standard).

Some decisions to stop treatment may be more tourbling and legally problematic as for example when there is a conflict among family members, or when there are no family members or appropriate surrogate decisionmakers available at all. Decisions perceived as efforts to limit the use of resources will be considered more legally controversial.

As with other termination of treatment decisions, certain steps should be followed to ensure that decisions are legally acceptably from a procedural standpoint. A discussion of procedures that are both ethically and legally acceptable can be found in the Hastings Center Guidelines [21]. Among the more important steps to follow, thorough documentation of all relevant circumstances is critical. The more complex and controversial the decision, the more documentation there should be. Also, formal written policies at the institutional level are of great value and the documentation in individual cases should note that practices in individual cases are in accordance with institutional policies.

Termination of treatment decisions are easier and less legally problematic when they are carried out in accordance with the patient's own wishes, expressed prior to incompetency. Patients should be encouraged to express what their wishes would be should this situation arise. Efforts to designate appropriate surrogate decisionmakers should be commonplace, even when patients are relatively healthy, and the benefits of dialysis clearly outweigh any burdens. Health care providers, especially physicians, should become much more comfortable with discussing these decisions with patients and family far in advance of deteriorating health and impending incompetency and decisions to continue or discontinue dialysis should be part of an overall treatment plan reached through interdisciplinary care conferences and extensive discussions with all involved. Even though the patient is the central focus of these decisions, there should be an attempt to arrive at consensual decisionmaking. There also should be far greater emphasis (especially for dialysis) on the moral and legal legitimacy of stopping treatment rather than withholding treatment in the first place. Thus, the patient is given every opportunity to benefit from a dialysis program without fearing that he or she will become a prisoner of an unthinking, uncaring medical system that lacks the moral courage to stop treatment when it is no longer of value.

In the final analysis, common sense and humane compassionate care consistent with current medical and ethical standards will almost always be legally acceptable. All discussions concerning what is legally acceptable should start with what makes the most sense and is most proper from an ethical standpoint. Good law follows good medicine and good ethics, not the reverse.

References

1. Meisel A. The right to die, 1990 Supplement. New York: Wiley Law Publications; 1990.
2. Lynn J, Glover J. Ethical decision-making in enteral nutrition. In Rombeau P, Coldwell MD (eds): Enteral and tube feeding, 2nd edition. Philadelphia: WB Saunders 1990: 575–86.
3. National Center for State Courts Life-sustaining medical treatment: Helping the courts decide. (Unpublished; final report to be released in 1991).
4. Society for the Right to Die. Legislation backgrounder. 1990.
5. Right-to-die case and statutory citations: State-by-state listing. News from Society for the Right to Die 1990, August.
6. Tube feeding laws in the United States. Society for the Right to Die Newsletter. New York; 15 October 1989.
7. Child abuse and neglect prevention and treatment, 45 C.F.R. Sections 1340. 1–1340. 20; 1986.
8. Weir RF, Gostin L. Decisions to abate life-sustaining treatment for nonautonomous patients. JAMA 1990; 264; 1846–52.
9. In re Conroy, 98 N.J. 321, 486 A.2d 1209; 1985.
10. Rhoden N. How should we view the incompetent? Law, Medicine & Health Care 1989; 17: 260–5.
11. In re Hier, 18 Mass. App. 200, 464 N.E. 2d 959; 1984. rev. denied, 392 Mass. 1102, 465 N.E.2d 261; 1984.
12. In re Jobes, 108 H. J. 394, 529 A.2d 434; 1987.
13. Corbett v. D'Alessandro, 487 So. 2d 368 (Fla. Dist. Ct. App.), review denied, 492 So. 2d 1331; Fla. 1986.
14. Brophy v. New England Sinai Hosp., Inc., 398 Mass. 417, 497 N.E.2d 626; 1986.
15. In re Peter, 108 N.J. 365, 529 A.2d 419; 1987.
16. Delio v. Westchester County Medical Center, 129 A.D.2d 1, 516 N.Y.S.2d 766; 1987.
17. In re Gardner, 534 A.2d 947; Me. 1987.
18. Gray V. Romeo, 697 F. Supp. 580; D.R.I. 1988.
19. McConnell V. Beverly Enterprises-Connecticut, Inc., 209 Conn. 692, 553 A.2d 596; 1989.
20. Deciding to forego life-sustaining treatment. Washington, DC: President's Commission for the Study of Ethical Problems in Medicine; 1983.
21. Guidelines on the termination of life-sustaining treatment and the care of the dying. Briarcliff Manor, NY: The Hastings Center; 1987.
22. Life-sustaining technologies and the elderly. Washington, DC: Office of Technology Assessment; 1987.
23. See amicus curiae briefs filed to the U.S. Supreme Court on behalf of petitioners in *Cruzan*: American Medical Association, American College of Surgeons, American Academy of Neurology, American Academy of Family Physicians, American Association of Neurological Surgeons, American Medical Women's Association, American Nurses Association, American Association of Nurse Attorneys, American College of Physicians, American Hospital Association, American Geriatrics Society, National Hospice Organization, Society for Critical Care Medicine.

142

24. Rhoden NK. Litigating life and death. Harvard Law Review 1988; 102: 375–446.
25. Eichner v. Dillon, 52 N.Y.2d 363, 420 N.E.2d 64, 438 N.Y.S.2d 266, cert. denied, 454 U.S. 858; 1981.
26. In re O'Connor 72, N.Y.2d 517, 531 N.E.2d 607, 534 N.Y.S.2d 866; 1988.
27. Cruzan v. Harmon, 760 S.W.2d 408 (Mo. 1988), cert. granted, 109 S. Ct. 3240; 1989.
28. In re Chad Eric Swan, 569 A.2d 1202; Me. 1990.
29. In re Torres, 357 N.W.2d 332; Minn. 1984.
30. The American Hospital Association, in its amicus curiae brief to the U.S. Supreme Court in *Cruzan*, stated that 70% of the 1.3 million patients who die in hospitals each year die after a decision to forgo life-sustaining treatment has been made. This number does not include patients who die at home or in nursing homes (1 Sept 1989, p. 3).
31. Superintendent of Belchertown State School v. Saikewicz, 373 Mass. 728, 370 N.E.2d 417; 1977.
32. Relman AS. The Saikewicz decision: Judges as physicians. N Engl J Med 1978 289: 508–9.
33. Weir RF. Abating treatment with critically ill patients: Ethical and legal limits to the medical prolongation of life. Oxford University Press; New York, 1989 pp. 116–7.
34. Liacos PJ. Dilemmas of dying. Medicolegal News 1979; 7 (29): 4–7.
35. Curran WJ. The Saikewicz decision. N Engl J Med 1978; 298: 499–500.
36. In re Spring, 380 Mass. 629, 405 N.E.2d 115; 1980 – at 121.
37. In re Lydia E. Hall Hosp., 116 Misc 2d 477, 455 N.Y.S.2d 706 (Sup. Ct. 1982).
38. Barron J. L.I. Hospital fights patient's plea to end lifesaving treatment. New York Times 1982 Oct 21:12.
39. In re Storar, 52. N.Y.2d 363, 420 N.E.2d 64, 438 N.Y.S.2d 266, cert. denied, 454 U.S. 858; 1981.
40. Gaylin W. A patient's rights must include power to refuse treatment. Minneapolis Star and Tribune 1982 Oct 29:16.
41. Sullivan R. Panel criticizes procedures for patients' consent for treatments. New York Times 1982 Oct 22:12.
42. Neu S, Kjellstrand CM. Stopping long-term dialysis: An empirical study of withdrawal of life-supporting treatment. N Engl J Med 1986; 314: 14–20.
43. In re Quinlan, 70 N.J. 10, 355 A.2d 647, cert. denied, 429 U.S. 922; 1976.
44. In re Dinnerstein, 6 Mass. App. 466, 380 N.E.2d 134; 1978.
45. Relman A. The *Saikewicz* decision: A medical viewpoint. Am J of Law & Med, 1978 4: 233–42.
46. Commissioner of Correction v. Myers, 399 N.E.2d 452; Mass, 1979.
47. Shapiro F. Personal communication, 29 November 1990.
48. New Mexico *ex rel.* Smith v. Fort, No. 14, 768; N.M. 1983.
49. Uniform Rights of the Terminally Ill Act [1985] 1–18, 9A U.L.A. 456; Supp. 1990.
50. Uniform Rights of the Terminally Ill Act [1989], 1–18, 9A U.L.A. 456; Supp. 1990.
51. In re Estate of Sidney Greenspan, No. 67903; Ill. Sup Ct. July, 1990.
52. State v. McAfee, 385 S.E.2d 651; GA. 1989.
53. Bouvia v. Superior Court (Glenchur), 179 Cal. App. 3d 1127, 225 Cal. Rptr. 297; 1986.
54. Hall MA. The malpractice standard under health care cost containment. Law, Medicine & Health Care 1989; 17: 347–55.
55. Brahams D. When is discontinuation of dialysis justified? Lancet 1985; 1(8421): 176–7.
56. Cruzan v. Director, Missouri Department of Health, 110 S. Ct. 2841; 1990.
57. Annas GJ. Nancy Cruzan and the right to die. N Engl J Med 1990; 323: 670–2.
58. In the estate of Nancy Beth Cruzan, Estate No. CB384-9P, Probate Division, Circuit Court of Jasper County, Missouri, Judge Charles E. Teel, Jr., July 27, 1988.
59. Annas GJ, Arnold B, Aroskar M *et al.* Bioethicists' statement on the U.S. Supreme Court's *Cruzan* decision. N Engl J Med 1990 323: 686–7.

11. An ethical analysis of stopping treatment

CARL M. KJELLSTRAND & JOHN B. DOSSETOR

*'We judge men by their actions, and we judge
actions by their results'.*

We live in a goal oriented society and this principle
has an immediate intuitive appeal.
However, intention rivals outcome in importance,
and although intention is more difficult to fathom and
weigh it is a necessary part of judging actions,
and thus men.

'We infer intention from actions'
(Samuel Johnson)

There are at least five different ethical systems that can be used when judging if an act is good or bad (Table I). None owes its origin to systems of divine revelation. None claims to be universal or overriding as the means to moral reasoning. We may look upon them all as perspectives of moral reasoning. A sixth system of value nihilism maintains that there is no such thing as a good or bad act, but it is all a matter of individual gut feeling. It is a useless system in the context of our analysis and will not be discussed further.

Table I

---

1. Kantian deontology – do what is one's duty, in recognition of the claims of others.
2. Utilitarianism or consequentialism – do what leads to the 'best' outcome, the maximum benefit for most people.
3. Virtue – To recognize that the personality traits of 'being' outrank outward acts of 'doing'.
4. Human mutual interdependency – To recognize that all are bound in a network of human relationships.
5. Existentialism – To acknowledge that each situation is unique, no principles are possible.

The first two theories provide ways by which acts may be judged; the third concentrates on cultivation of good traits of character which motivates right acts; the fourth is a fundamental ethic of human relationship; the fifth recognizes that a person's whole experience and responses are unique expressions of being which cannot be reduced to action principles or rules.

143

C. M. Kjellstrand and J. B. Dossetor (eds): Ethical Problems in Dialysis and Transplantation, 143–151.
© 1992 *Kluwer Academic Publishers. Printed in the Netherlands.*

Physicians, schooled for decades in empirical approach to difficult questions, often intuitively deny any value to normative research where the outcomes are analyzed so objectively [1, 2]. Some even believe that medical ethicists have only contributed to the damage of medical values. They believe that patients are ultimately hurt by ethicists who have confused the care givers; these ethicists are in fact responsible for warping the expectations of patients and relatives by the replacement of useful and practical medical norms and duties with abstract, unrealistic, hypothetical hair-splitting [3]. Others believe that technology has spawned so many new dilemmas that the threat posed to wise decision-making can only be counteracted by physicians being trained in biomedical ethics and by other disciplines being admitted to the decision-making process at the bedside [4].

Many moral choices are not between good and bad, but between bad and worse, as may be the case in certain ESRD patients when faced with the decision to discontinue or continue treatment. To some, continuing treatment appears like torture; to others, stopping therapy appears to be murder. Difficulties in drawing lines does not mean that lines should not be drawn. Aristotle discussed this, concluding: *'the lesser evil is reckoned a good in comparison with a greater evil, since the lesser evil is rather to be chosen than the greater, and what is worthy of choice is good and what is worthier of choice, a greater good'* [5].

I. Kantian deontology

Kant said *'I admire two things above everything else, the starry sky above me and the moral law within'*, and *'act only in such a way that you can also will that the maxim should become a universal law'* – the categorical imperative [6]. He believed that all 'moral agents' are endowed with a moral intuition that tells us what is right and what is wrong. To test that an action is moral we have to consider that our response to another's claim on us should become a rule which applies equally to us and to everyone, i.e. universally. Deontology claims that a rule for stopping treatment would only be ethically correct if it could be applied equally to all dialysis patients in the same situation. Thus, 'do not dialyze patients over 80' is unacceptable as a moral statement, as most careproviders would hold that it should not be applied, universally. However, a rule based which stated that 'all competent patients should be free to refuse dialysis when they perceive that burden outweighs benefit' would be acceptable as a universal moral precept.

It appears as if Kant summarized the great religions who put it differently but presented the same message: 'Do unto others as you would have them do unto you', with its important corollary 'Don't do unto others that which you would not want them to do unto you.'

II. Utilitarianism

The utilitarian principle is based on the philosophy of the 17th and 18th century, and is best characterized by Bentham and Mill. It has much to recommend it in its social application, often expressed as 'the maximum amount of benefit for the maximum number of individuals'. It is customary to recognize two forms of Utilitarianism: Act and Rule [7]. The former applies the principle of utility to individual acts, the latter applies the principle of utility to rules. For example, a rule which stated that one should not discriminate against the elderly would be acceptable to utilitarianism as it exemplifies the rule of non-discrimination and thus represents great benefit to all, including younger sections of the population. However, an act which denies dialysis treatment to an 84 year old with early Alzheimer's dementia, while acceptable to an act utilitarian might not be an acceptable decision to a deontologist or to a rule utilitarian.

Act utilitarianism in medical practice entails making a benefits and burdens balance sheet of the consequences of the act. Applied to medicine in general it appears to be detrimental to an individual patient's interests. From a societal point of view, it is always expensive to treat the old and the ill where the goals are often so limited, so such treatment would always carry little weight against society's perceived greater good were it not for the rule that it is in the interests of a benevolent and humane society to look after the elderly. Act utilitarianism, in medicine, may seem to be a tool for rationing resources. However, most utilitarians apply the system in respect to moral rules. Decisions made by deontology and rule utilitarianism are often the same, though the process of reasoning differs in each. We will discuss in a later chapter the practicalities of stopping treatment, and show that utilitarianism can be a very helpful system in analyses of the possible courses of action.

III. Virtue

The ethics of virtue receives little emphasis in modern biomedical ethics [8] though it was the basis for Aristotle's ethics system and is fundamental to the rational ethics of Aquinas. The crucial difference is that virtue appeals to the mental qualities or personality traits which motivate actions, in contrast to examination of acts as calls to duty under a particular categorical imperative or as justified by their consequences. It is possible to act in an outwardly kind and compassionate way towards persons while, in fact, not feeling well disposed or compassionate towards them in one's mind.

Because virtue ethics deals with mental or psychological dispositions and motivations it is much harder to assess than are actions. Despite this, in health care there are many calls for virtuous action which seem to extend beyond the claims or duty

or towards foreseeable good consequences. Examples of this would include: sentiments or feelings of genuinely shared grief; feelings of brotherly or sisterly love
towards patients; feelings of personal joy at patients' happiness; or, a willingness to
place patients' interests ahead of those of the caregiver.

These, and many more, are the components of character which are at the heart of
health care and we should not ignore them in relation to ethical behaviour.

IV. Human mutual interdependency

An ethic which recognizes the interrelationship of all human beings – in health care:
patients, physicians, nurses, pharmacists, technicians and administrators, alike – has
many advocates. Some of the strongest proponents are feminist philosophers such as
Carol Gilligan [9] and Annette Baier [10]. They point out that the North American
systems of bioethics, based on the four cardinal principles, especially autonomy
(*vide infra*) is built idealistically on concepts of 'moral agents' who are equal, with
equal rights. In reality, much of life consists of interactions between individuals who
are not equal, who cannot equally express their autonomy, who may not be good
decision-makers, who do not thrive on autonomous independence, or who cannot
readily defend themselves against those who confront them. The proponents of the
ethic of mutual interdependency – the caring perspective – see it as superior to and
extending beyond that of an autonomy based ethic – the rights perspective – even
though it may be unsuitable for development into principles and rules.

Such an ethic has much to offer the difficult issues in health care. Physicians,
armed with the symbolism of stethoscope, white coat and the distance across the
polished mahogany desk, subconsciously separate themselves from patients. The
technology of diagnostic testing augments this distancing. Whilst all this may still
be compatible with the cardinal principles and rules of deontologic or utilitarian
ethics, physicians and other caregivers should also recognize their patients' claim
for dependency upon them, of the need to exercise humanity, empathy and compas-
sion towards them, or the patients' desire for caregivers to become involved with
them as individuals. This of course is the complete antipathy of 'here are the facts,
the complications, the prognostic outcomes, go and think about it and come back
with your decision'.

V. Existentialism

Existentialism, as best expressed by the writings of Kirkegaard and Sartres, states
that many morally complicated situations are so intricate that overriding principles
are not possible or necessary [11]. Thus, each patient's problems, personality, background, and treatment circumstances are so varied that each decision is unique and
best solved isolated from others. Physicians in their resistance to have their actions

judged, appear to intuitively like this system best. However, the danger of existentialism is that it leads only in *ad hoc* decisions and takes away any logical analysis of the decision to stop or continue. Although it is useful to make an overall emotional analysis of the situation a patient is in, as we will describe later in the practicalities of stopping dialysis, existentialism, by saying that things are often complicated and confusing, allows no contemplation of the issue and seems to be of little help.

VI. The process of ethical decision-making

As mentioned earlier, decision-making is usually not able to rest on one or other of these five theoretical approaches. In practice, while one trusts that one's motivation is compatible with and sensitive to the principles of virtue, while one hopes that an awareness of our human mutual interdependency enlightens all our dealings with others, and while one also wishes to treat each patient as unique in an existentialist way, one is forced to conduct an analysis of situations according to the claims of duty and the likely consequences of action. This is an essential part of decision-making.

The principles of bioethics can be used in relation to any of these five bioethics perspectives, but the four main principles coupled with the duty of patient advocacy, as outlined in Chapter 4 previously, form the accepted basis for deontologic and utilitarian ethics analysis. We have returned to their consideration after going through other ethical theories because of their practical value, despite their derivation from the 'rights'-based approach to problems in biomedical ethics. In so doing we do not wish to ignore the ethic of mutual interdependency between unequals with varying degrees of vulnerability.

What then are the principles of bioethics and what is the role of emotion, or feelings, in applying them? The principles are:

1. Beneficence – do good, respect life.
2. Patient autonomy – the patient in control.
3. Non-maleficence – do not harm, avoid harm.
4. Distributive Justice – to each according to need.
5. The duty of advocacy.

Some argue that beneficence can be interpreted as prolonging life at all costs, or respecting the sanctity of life. If adopted as an absolute value this overrides the other principles. If one accepts this ranking, terminating therapy to let a patient die is always bad even when requested by patients or their surrogates. Those holding this view of beneficence as equal to the sanctity of life maintain that a physician who participates in stopping dialysis, has violated the highest ethical maxim a physician can have. When arguing along this line and when the outcome is invariably death, some philosophers such as Anscombe and Dolan [12, 13] equate stopping treatment with murder. Anscomb defines murder as 'the intentional killing of the innocent', though whether she would maintain this stance if the innocent person and family request it, is less clear. She further accepts that standing passively by and refusing to prevent death from occurring can be morally equal to actively killing someone. She quotes St. Aquinas: 'It was both possible and necessary for the agent to act and he did not'.

Most people, however, are not so absolutist and see the principle of beneficence as respect for life, respect for persons, and doing good, however that may be best conceived. Beneficence is perceived by Pellegrino [14] as overarching and inclusive of the principle of respect for patient autonomy. To such ethicists beneficence would not be served by prolonging life at all costs. Indeed, in those situations where patient and family plead for death by allowing discontinuation of treatment, e.g. by discontinuation of dialysis, beneficence may well be served. Further, failing to do so might well be interpreted as contravention of the principle of non-maleficence.

Beneficence does not always trump all other considerations. In different situations the three principles will rank differently. In the emergency room one violates the autonomy of the suicide victim by lavaging the stomach, because beneficence and the avoidance of maleficence override autonomy. In the aged dialysis patient who has calmly contemplated his situation and come to the conclusion that the sum of his diseases is a misfortune that no longer makes life worth living, one obeys his wishes and stops dialysis in order to let him die, after first ruling out psychiatric and underlying correctible psychosomatic illnesses. In this conclusion, respect for autonomy overrides the 'absolutist' notion of beneficence. When patients cannot decide for themselves one listens to the family, who know the individual best and jointly come to consensus – family, nurses and physicians together – on that course of action which they believe best reflects the patient's own will.

J. Rachels [13] contends that active euthanasia is sometimes a greater good than passive euthanasia (stopping treatment) and that there is no moral difference between active and passive euthanasia. Why not inject potassium chloride into the competent patient who does not want to continue dialysis? Obviously this will cause cardiac arrest and death, but so will stopping dialysis which also results in hyperpotassemia and cardiac arrest. The acts, he argues, are morally equivalent but to take positive action may be more beneficent. The end is identical, the means to the end are similar, therefore why should one let the patient suffer the pain and the horror of expecting his demise over many days, when it can be compressed into seconds or minutes? Rachels uses examples of patients with Downs syndrome needing complicated operations that one declines to do, or those dying of incurable cancer with terrible untreatable pain who suffer interminably. Rachels' examples are realistic and are similar to those encountered by dialysis physicians. Such patients cause severe moral and emotional problems for those caring for them.

Arguments against these who equate active and passive euthanasia are as follows:

1. Physicians should never mentally will the death of patients, though they may accede to competent patients' refusal of treatment which may lead to death. Physicians are not the harbingers of death but must remain dedicated to preserving life and relief of suffering and serving patient autonomy. Active killing, even on request, is not within that definition [16]. There are limits, moral and legal, to the physician role, and actively helping a death is beyond that limit, in our view.

2. All who face this dilemma must experience an 'existentialistic' gut feeling about the enormous moral difference between deliberately, actively, injecting a substance to kill and that of turning off a respirator or discontinuing dialysis. To be unable to give a rational ethical explanation for this gut feeling is not enough to discredit its validity, however. It is reflected in legal practice in various nations. Those who indulge in mercy killing are often prosecuted for murder, though admittedly few are convicted or severely punished. On the other hand, no physician has been convicted of murder for stopping or withdrawing treatment, although this is a very common practice [17–20].

3. To kill in mercy, while understandable, would imperil society's trust in physicians. The old and sick will fear hospitals as places where they might be killed, especially as economic pressures grow on the provision of expensive life prolonging technologies.

4. Active euthanasia has the pragmatic difficulty of its control and the detection of possible abuse.

The Netherlands now allows physicians to actively kill competent consenting patients – the law of homicide has been made non-prosecutable in medical situations of this sort. The conditions are carefully defined. Several thousand such killings are said to occur yearly and are openly admitted. It is claimed, and this can be used in argument against point #3 above, that this has not led to any widespread fears or mistrust in patients who have been referred to hospitals [21], it cannot be used as a counter argument against point #2 as it remains illegal, but condoned.

Weighing the arguments for and against the two extremes, we believe a strong argument and defense can be made for the middle ground. 'Yes', one is allowed to stop treatment to let patients die but 'No!', no-one is permitted to actively kill them.

The principles of beneficence, non-maleficence and respect for patient autonomy weigh differently in different cases. What is the role of feelings, or emotion, in these decisions? What is the *moral authority* of such a gut feeling, as expressed in #2 above?

In the history of ethics the role played by our emotions, in contrast to rationality or reason, per se, has long been controversial. Of various schools of thought, that which has the most appeal is that which claims that rationality *per se* does not give one the answer. Rationality only provides the reasoned analysis, but does not necessarily inform the actual decision. The decision, it seems to us, stems from the individual's emotional commitment to a given solution (based on the overt rationality of the case in point, together with the subconscious imprint of previous experience gathered over a lifetime – another name for intuition, perhaps). Committing oneself to a decision has, so it would seem, a strong emotional element, a definite feeling. This is how one would justify the statement concerning 'gut feeling', in #2 above. This component of decision-making has been emphasized by Callahan [22] as follows: 'Emotions energize the ethical quest. A good case can be made that what is specifically moral about moral thinking, what gives it its imperative "oughtness", is personal emotional investment. When emotion infuses an evaluative judgement, it is transformed into a prescriptive moral judgement of what ought to be done'.

A similar process: analysis leading, at the final step, to a decision based on emotion may be illustrated by the following tale. The Persian Emperor Xerxes, when asked the difference between 'good' and 'bad' invited two tribes to explain how they dealt with their elderly, after death. One tribe ate them, the other burned them. Each tribe was equally horrified by the other's approach. Their distaste for the other's customs was visceral. Eating the dead was a gross abomination to one tribe, burning them a horrible waste of their wisdom to the other. Although there are undeniable profound cultural practices between these two tribes they are due to differences in the emotional commitment to two different sets of cultural values – to eat, or to incinerate, based on their collective feelings about the matter. Yet, they both clearly shared an important overarching principle – veneration for the dead.

Stopping dialysis is not murder, but may be the lesser of evils and therefore a greater good. There is no problem with elevating the act of stopping treatment, under the conditions we have defined, to becoming a universal law. Indeed, as mentioned above, it may also be acceptable under rule utilitarianism.

VII. Summary

There are five theoretical perspectives to ethical analysis of stopping or continuing dialysis: deontology, utilitarianism, virtue, mutual interdependency, and existentialism.

Of these, deontology based on the concept of duty and the constraints of the categorical (unconditional) moral imperative appears to be the better of the two systems which depend on the analysis of actions. The other three systems all have merit and need to be borne in mind in such a difficult subject as acceding to the willed death of an individual patient.

To extremists who interpret deontology as prohibiting cessation of treatment under any circumstances, the correct deontological answer would be that none of the three moral principles of beneficence, non-maleficence and autonomy always trumps the others. To those who hold the viewpoint that active euthanasia is morally permissible, our rejoinder would be that most people would not like to see such a principle universalized, and therefore the practice cannot be defended from the deontological point of view. It is noted that rational analysis displays the part played by principles and rules in decisions of this sort, but this process alone may not lead to a solution. In the final step one finds such sentiments as 'gut feeling' or 'firm conviction' or 'belief' (unsubstantiated by rationality). It is this component which we have termed the element of emotion, or of feelings, in decision-making. It is an indispensable last step, but must be preceded by the rigorous exercise of reason.

References

1. Kass LR. Ethical dilemmas in the care of the ill, part 1. JAMA 1980; 244: 1811–6.
2. Kass LR. Ethical dilemmas in the care of the ill, Part 2. JAMA 1980; 244; –1946–9.
3. Clements CD, Sider RC. Medical ethics' assault on medical values. JAMA 1983; 250: 2011.
4. Rothman DJ. Strangers at the bedside: A history of how law and bioethics transformed medical decision making. Basic Books, Inc. 1991.
5. Ross D. The Nichomachean ethics of Aristotle, Book V. Oxford Univ. Press, 1961.
6. Kant I. Groundwork of the metaphysic of morals. Patton HJ (ed). Harper Torchbooks/Academy Library, New York, 1964.
7. Beauchamp TL, Childress JF. Principles of biomedical ethics. Oxford Univ. Press 1989, chapter 2.
8. Beauchamp TL, Childress JF. Principles of biomedical ethics. Oxford Univ. Press, 3rd edition, 1989, chapter 8.
9. Gilligan Carol, Remapping the Moral Domain: New images of self in relationship, In Gilligan C, Ward JV, Taylor JM (eds): Mapping the Moral Domain. Harvard Univ. Press, 1988, pp. 3–20.
10. Baier, Annette C. The need for more than justice. In Hanen M, Niehlsen K (ed): Science, morality & feminist theory. Canadian J Philosophy. 1987; (Supp.) 13: 41–56.
11. Kirkegaard S, Ross SL (ed): Either/Or Harper & Row, New York; 1986.
12. Anscombe GEM. Murder and the morality of euthanasia: some philosophical considerations. In: Euthanasia and clinical practice, chapter 3. The Linacre Centre, London; 1982.
13. Dolan JM. Lethal medicine. Trans Am Soc Artif Intern Organs 1986; 32: 672–5.
14. Pellegrino ED. Withholding and withdrawing treatments: ethics at the bedside. Clinical Neurosurgery 1989; 35: 164–84.
15. Rachels J Active and passive euthanasia. N Engl J Med 1973; 292: 78–80.; and Trans Am Soc Artif Intern Organs 1986; 32: 638–87, Also, The end of life: Euthanasi and morality Oxford Univ. Press; 1986
16. Dossetor JB. Withdrawal of treatment: is it ever justifiable? Humane Medicine 1991; 7(3): 217–21.
17. Neu S, Kjellstrand CM. Stopping long-term dialysis. An empirical study of withdrawal of life-supporting treatment. New Eng J Med 1986; 314: 14–20.
18. Port FK, Wolf RA, Hawthorne VM et al. Discontinuation of dialysis therapy as a cause of death. Am J Nephrol 1989; 9: 145–9.
19. Wehle B, Ahlmen J. Prudent withdrawal of chronic dialysis treatment. Scand J Urol Nephrol Suppl 1990; 131: 47–8.
20. Hirsch DJ. Death from dialysis termination. Nephrol Dial Transplant 1989; 4: 41–4.
21. Pence GE. Do not go slowly into that Dark Night: mercy killing in Holland. Am J Med 1988; xxx: 139–41.
22. Callahan S. The role of emotion in ethical decision-making. Hastings Center Report June/July 1988: 9–14.

PART FOUR

Different views from different countries

12. A perspective on reality

Almost two decades since the first successful renal transplant was performed in India international interest in the transplant scene here has been evoked by the extensive use of paid living donors as a source of kidneys. Hindu society is very complex and often contradictory and to quote Pallis [1]: "A common thread unites the most abstract philosophical speculations, and a childish belief in ghosts; a deep respect for non-violence, and the bloodiness of sarcrificial rituals; extreme asceticism, and the sexual aspect of Tantric worship." So it is not surprising that few people have the kind of social abhorrence attached to paid donations of organs as in affluent occidental societies.

Consider the fate of any one of sixty to eighty thousand new cases of End-Stage Renal Disease (hereafter called ESRD) that are anticipated in India each year. What are their chances of survival? Consider these facts:

1. No cadaver donor program is in existence in the country.
2. Other than in exceptional circumstances long term hemodialysis as a practical alternative in India is almost impossible to achieve.
   2.1 In a survey done by Parry and Co. [2] and Susruta Agencies [3] in 1989, only 640 hemodialysis machines were found to exist in this country. Even if the number has doubled in the past few months the total is still woefully inadequate.
   2.2 The perennial unreliability of power and water supply and the difficulty in the maintenance of these machines limits hemodialysis facilities to the major cities of India, thus disrupting the lives of families of hundreds of patients who are forced to move to these cities for dialysis.
   2.3 Long term survival rates on hemodialysis in India are poor. No figures are available but it is our educated guess that it is below 10–15% three year survival (unless someone proves the contrary to us, against a proven 74% three-year patient survival rate after unrelated live donor transplantation). [4]
   2.4 On the economic level, there are few if any long term state aided or insurance funded programs for chronic hemodialysis. Nearly all dialyses and transplantations are confined to the private sector whose 'raison d'être' is

C. M. Kjellstrand and J. B. Dossetor (eds): Ethical Problems in Dialysis and Transplantation, 155–161.
© 1992 *Kluwer Academic Publishers. Printed in the Netherlands.*

156

profit. If monetary gain were the only consideration, more money could be made effortlessly by dialysis.

In our judgement, the only chance of long term survival for ESRD patients is a living donor transplant.

Let us digress at this point to consider a possible classification of all potential donors, as shown in Table 1.

Table 1.

A. *Cadaver*

    A.1 *The 'opting-in' cadaver donor*
The donor who previously voluntarily signed a donor card. His gift of organs is voluntary, universal, anonymous and posthumous, and is the only truly altruistic form of donation.

    A.2 *Consent from next-of-kin for retrieval of cadaveric organs*
This is always tempered by the fact that more people would donate other people's organs than their own.

    A.3 *The 'opting-out' and legislation for cadaver donor*
This is possible only if legislation is brought in to permit removal of cadaveric organs without consent of the family of the deceased. In our minds this would be unacceptable as the state would be usurping the rights of the deceased individual's family.

B. *Living*
    B.1 *Genetic*
        a) *For love*
The gift is specific for the recipient. The donor is emotionally vulnerable. Failure of such grafts gives emotional trauma to the donor (Shastry JCM, pers. comm.)

        b) *Concealed coerced consent*
In male dominated Hindu society, the women in the family are invariably emotionally and socially vulnerable, and this fact becomes obvious when genetically related donor lists are scrutinized.

        c) *Involving exchange of money or property*
In many intra-familial kidney donations the donor probably benefits financially, as well. Statistics for this are not available.

    B.2 *Non-genetic*
        a) *Emotionally related donors*
This may be from either a spouse or a close friend. Spousal donations particularly from the wife, in India, are probably coerced except where marriage has lasted for at least ten years. In India, marriages are often arranged to poor women to acquire a kidney.

        b) *Paid donors*
          (i) *'Rewarded gifting'*: Acceptable practices characterized by no involvement of middlemen; institutionalized control; full informed consent and guaranteed follow up of donors.
          (ii) *'Rampant commercialization'*: Unacceptable practices; involvement of touts, inadequate consent, no follow up, surgical operations being performed in nursing homes ill-equipped for these operations, etc.

From our experience we believe that about 40% of genetically related donors are subtly coerced, or stand to obtain monetary benefit. Medicine has no difficulty accepting this with the explanation "Exchange of money is within the scope of family ethics". But do not need-based family ethics in a way reflect social values and social acceptability? Can we as physicians stand idly by, and allow patients to die, when we have the means at hand to save their lives without causing significant harm to anyone?

When one considers any live donor transplantation the Hippocratic doctrine of *'primum non nocere'* is transgressed. Under such circumstances, is payment of money to a willing, informed adult so unethical or immoral that it alone decides whether patients should be allowed to live or die? It seems ironic that all agents involved in the transplantation process are financially benefitted except the donor who is excluded on the grounds that payment would be immoral or unethical! Having resolved that paid donation is not unethical in itself, what are the other controversial aspects of such practice?

I. Donor vulnerability

No act of organ donation is entirely free from clinical risk and therefore it is essential that consent should be free, informed and voluntary. Yet, when psychological and emotional pressures that must fall on the live related donor are considered, this assumption fails [5]. Although this pressure differs vastly from the pressure of financial inducement, it is nonetheless pressure; pressure which is acutely intensified when alternate modalities of treatment are non-existent, as in India. In real life situations decisions are based on need and not on abstract philosophies; therefore it is mutual need and lack of alternatives that bring donor and recipient together. Exploitation only occurs when advantage is taken of either the donor or the recipient, but when fair and adequate compensation is made, such exploitation ceases to exist. So for any form of living donor transplantation some form of external coercion is inevitable.

II. Donor motivation

If financial need alone was the only reason for unrelated live donation, potential donor lists would be filled from the ranks of the destitute, but scrutiny of our donor lists reveals three major groups of donors: a) single young men with stable family backgrounds who are the head of a family and are directly responsible for the social and financial welfare of their family; b) widowed or abandoned women who have similarly been left with responsibility for their children; and c) well-established family units in which the couple are in their twenties or thirties with completed families.

True, all of them have financial needs. Needs that could be met by criminal or other unsocial activity, but the choice to sell and preserve one's self-respect lies in the Hindu ethos of the paramountcy of performing one's duties and fulfilling obligations – dharma. How else can one explain the fact that in no other society will a young man or mother sell their kidney for performing the marriage of their sisters or daughters, or for that matter to settle family debts or to secure the future of their minor children? The act of sacrifice in performing one's dharma ennobles the donor rather than degrading him. The increase in individuals' self-esteem and emotional benefit is considerable. In spite of criticism in the press [6] new donors come forward after seeing the improved quality of life and self-esteem of past donors. In such circumstances perhaps the most difficult and painful decision in unrelated live donor selection process is finding an otherwise healthy donor unfit on the grounds of anatomically poor renal vasculature.

III. Donor follow-up

Whatever inducements are offered, donor compliance for follow-up is poor and is often difficult to enforce. Donors want their financial compensation immediately and occasionally request that the money be kept aside for their medical insurance payments. Any form of annuity payment is rarely acceptable to the donor. Often donors leave the city and return to their rural homes to start life again and few leave forwarding addresses. Not that this state of affairs is confined to the paid donors alone. From 500 letters sent to *related* donors to come for follow-up at the Christian Medical College, Vellore, India, only 50 returned for medical re-examination (Shastry JCM, pers. comm.). The follow-up at our centre has been equally dismal. From the 20% or so of donors who have been seen in follow-up, certain conclusions can be drawn:

(a) *Medical*: No serious problems have been attributed to the nephrectomy. Several cases of incisional hernia and varicocele have needed surgical correction. The majority of conditions have been unrelated to previous nephrectomy, such as injuries, tropical infections and gastroenteritis.
(b) *Social*: Here again only limited data is available. To suggest that a poor donor will not be able to manage his new found resources is to suggest that the poor should be allowed to remain in their poverty. There is no doubt that a few will waste their financial reward but many have definitely improved their standard of living and few have regretted their decision to donate. We have gradually learned to tailor out donor selection process so that optimum social benefit is derived. The emotional benefit derived by these donors has already been alluded to.

It must be remembered by all those involved in paid organ donation that the minute an incision is made in the donor all the obligations and responsibilities of the doctor/patient relationship are automatically conferred on the donor and assumed by the practitioner.

IV. Disincentive to live related donor transplantation

Patients who have truly voluntary genetically related donors rarely opt out to have paid donor transplantation. The main objectors are parents who refuse donation from their young unmarried offspring. In spite of the availability of paid donors, the number of live related transplantations done in the three major transplant centres in Tamil Nadu State of India have actually been on the increase. In our centre we have the certain knowledge that genetically related donors are truly voluntary, as patients do have alternate means for transplantation.

V. Disincentive for cadaver transplantation

In an article entitled "Needed, a campaign for cadaver donations", M.K. Mani [7] states that he opposes the use of paid donations because this removes the pressure which would otherwise be exerted on the government by the rich and the influential to initiate a cadaver transplant program. There is no doubt that the ideal solution would be a cadaver donor program, but to transfer the onus of getting a cadaver program going by these unfortunates, who have more serious problems on their hands, is a serious dereliction of duty of those in the medical profession who should be at the vanguard of such endeavours. If the argument is that the government should be pressured by these patients to provide a cadaver program, how much more effective the pressure would be if *all* living donor transplantation were stopped till a cadaver program is started. After all, from a statistical viewpoint, the addition of about 750 to 1000 (assumed annual number of live related donor transplantations in India) to the already 60–80,000 who will die of ESRD for want of any treatment is insignificant.

It must also be remembered that, as yet, there are no legal and other infrastructural and logistical aspects for a national transplant program in place. Our nation, with its high indebtedness, can scarcely afford such a program when so many other priorities have to be attended to. Furthermore, no facilities exist for state-aided maintenance of a large number of patients on chronic hemodialysis while awaiting cadaver transplantation.

VI. Victimization of the poor by the rich

The act of organ donation is always a two-way street – almost like the quality of mercy. In the genetically related, the donor is emotionally vulnerable and the act of donation gives the satisfaction of seeing a loved one live. The paid donor is financially vulnerable, but his act achieves two objectives, (i) the kidney may have helped a patient to live, and, (ii) substantial emotional benefit is derived from having fulfilled family duties and obligations. In a way there has been a mutual transfer of health in the totality of its meaning.

VII. Permitting paid organ donations will lead to medical, commercial and social malpractices

Whenever demand exceeds supply, it is in the nature and ingenuity of man that the demand side will prevail. Under the circumstances, the people and not the system will determine whether the system works for the good or the bad. Legalizing and regulating the activity of paid organ donation, till such time alternate methods of treatment are made available, is the best insurance against the development of a blackmarket in organs.

VIII. Paid organ donation will remain a service for the rich

From the economic point of view, as far as transplantation or dialysis is concerned, nothing is free as 90% of the activity is in the private sector. Further, at our centre if one computes the cost of a live unrelated donor transplant maintained for two years, it would be less than the cost of purchasing a hemodialysis machine and running it for the same period. Also, scrutiny of our lists of recipients shows that only a small proportion of patients are drawn from the ranks of the rich. Large numbers of patients have been referred and paid for by the defence services and persons related to the Government of India, besides private sector companies. A good number of these patients also receive financial aid from charitable institutions, the general public, the Prime Minister's and Chief Minister's relief funds and the Governor's and President's discretionary funds.

Having argued that paid organ donation is an acceptable modality of treatment of ESRD in India and that it can be suitably controlled and monitored, we have devised and practised such a program [8, 9], at the Pandalai Cardio Thoracic Foundation and the Guest Hospital, Madras. From our experience of over 500 such transplants we have drawn the following conclusions:

1. The system can work to meet the special medico-socio-economic conditions prevailing in India and render justice to all parties concerned.
2. The attendant evils of rampant commercialization can be eliminated by institutionalizing the donor selection process and keeping all financial transactions above board.
3. The results of such controlled transplantations are good [10].

4. If state-aided autonomous bodies are appointed to oversee the process in recognized institutions and to screen potential recipients for financial aid, all patients can have access to this program depending on their intrinsic medical indication.

Undertaking to perform a paid organ transplant is not an easy decision. That it has to be considered at all as a modality of treatment is a reflection of the relentless progress of modern medicine and increasing expectation of dying patients, against a background of disparate socio-economic conditions. Its social acceptance is linked to the fact that it is commendable to make personal sacrifice in the pursuit of performance of one's duties. Provided the care of the donor in all respects can be guaranteed, paid organ donation is an acceptable alternative in India as has been confirmed by our experience and those of independent observers from the profession [11] and media [12].

What lessons are there then for the developed world in all this? The cadaver program has not been able to provide for the progressive increase in the demand for donor organs. Further advances in immunosuppressive regimens is going to increase the safety and long-term results of transplantation, and patients' expectations will be heightened. With soaring medical costs and shrinking health budgets few countries can afford to keep all patients indefinitely on chronic dialysis. When availability of all methods of treatment becomes limited, who decides which patient will be allowed to die? When cadaver organs become scarce who will have the priority access to them – the rich, the young, the white or the male? When the state is unable to provide should not the individual be allowed to provide for himself? Does the answer lie in some form of 'rewarded gifting'? Ultimately societies have to decide this question for themselves.

References

1. Pallis. Permission to quote requested.
2. Parry and Co. 1988: Market survey.
3. Susruta Agencies. 1988: Market survey.
4. Daar A, Sells R. On behalf of the Ethical Committee of the Transplantation Society, to the President and Council of the Transplantation Society; 1989: p. 16.
5. Martyn Evans. Organ donations should not be restricted to relatives. J Med Ethics 1989; 15: 17–20.
6. Muthuramalingam, Sivaram, Vallava. Beware of doctors. Nakkiran, June 23, 1990.
7. Mani MK. Needed; a campaign for cadaver donations. The Hindu, August 19, 1990; p. 19.
8. Reddy KC, Thiagarajan CM, Shunmugasundaram D. *et. al*. Unconventional renal transplantation in India. Transplant Proc 1990; 22 (3) (June): 912–4.
9. Thiagarajan CM, Reddy KC, Shunmugasundaram D. *et al*. Unconventional renal transplantation in India. Transplant Proc 1990; 11 (3) (June): 912–4.
10. Daar A, Sells R, 1989: *ibid*, p. 16.
11. Daar A, Sells, R, 1989; *ibid*, p. 17.
12. Raj Chengappa. The organs bazaar. India Today, July 31, 1990 pp. 60–7.

13. The argument against the unrelated live donor

M.K. MANI

The organ most often transplanted is the blood. The demand for blood in India is extremely large, and for years, blood banks made little effort to encourage voluntary donations. It was too much trouble to persuade people to donate blood, and too easy to find needy persons who were happy to give this renewable commodity and collect a little pocket money. With developments in surgery, and the growth of cardiothoracic surgical units which called for large amounts of blood of specific types, it became more difficult for blood banks to meet the demand. Some of them made efforts to inform the public of the need, and to identify people with uncommon blood groups who could be called on to donate blood when their particular group was wanted. This called for the expenditure of considerable time and energy, which was not always forthcoming, from the blood bank staff.

Many blood banks gratefully accepted the help of some 'social workers' who brought in donors. Many of the poor who inhabit the streets of our big cities would gladly sell their blood but were unaware of the possibility. They were ready to part with a fraction of their remuneration as a commission to the person who told them about it. The entrepreneurial spirit led to the development of a system of brokers who located the donors, brought them to the hospital, and collected a commission either from the blood bank or from the donor. This has become a recognized profession.

The system works well, but there are many grave dangers associated with it. Both the broker and the donor have a vested interest in the sale of blood, and therefore will not inform the blood bank of any reasons why that person's blood should not be used. The broker coaches the donor to suppress information about any illness which might make his blood unacceptable, and about recent donations elsewhere. Thus, this system becomes a hazard both to the donor and to the community. However, it is a fact of life.

Since the price paid for the product is quite small, the disadvantage to the ambitious broker is the limited money he can earn by the sale of blood. He must leave enough for the seller to serve as an adequate incentive. The advent of renal transplantation in India has been a godsend to this profession. The sums paid for a kidney are infinitely larger than for blood, so many brokers diversified into this new product. The principles of the trade remain the same.

C. M. Kjellstrand and J. B. Dossetor (eds): Ethical Problems in Dialysis and Transplantation, 163–168.
© 1992 *Kluwer Academic Publishers. Printed in the Netherlands.*

Who are the donors of these organs? Many patients who decide to take an unrelated donor transplant advertise in the press, and thus obtain their kidney. A lady in one of India's richest industrial families published two column advertisements running the length of the entire page in a number of the country's leading newspapers. It is believed that the response was in tens of thousands. An immunologist was then hired to go to major cities in the country where these potential donors had been screened and collected, and suitable candidates were tissue typed, until finally an identical donor was found. Patient and donor then went overseas to complete the transaction. I understand the transplant has been a success.

The average patient does not have the funds for this sort of advertising campaign, and satisfies himself or herself with a smaller advertisement. The chance of this being seen by the ultimate donor himself is small, but the brokers who are on the look-out for such business opportunities do spot them and parade their wares before the buyer. I have been told by some that the negotiations are often unpleasant and that the broker is likely to be persistent and to make a nuisance of himself. Obviously, many would rather avoid this aspect.

Many would-be donors who wish to sell their kidneys write to nephrologists at the leading hospitals. I have received many of these letters. There are two standard formats. In one, the writer says he would like to help suffering humanity by donating one kidney to some unfortunate patient, and would like to do it free, but needs to protect his family against any misfortune to himself and therefore requires a sum, usually considerable, to be paid in advance. Others are more honest, and tell of their own financial misfortunes and the urgency to raise funds, and therefore say they are constrained to sell their organs. I know some nephrologists who keep these letters on file and make them available to their patients.

However, the donors of the majority of transplants done today are not located in this manner. They come from the pavements of the cities, and are often youths who have come from villages and small towns to find jobs, but have been unsuccessful and are now desperate. Hunger and disease make them eager to obtain some money by any means, but also make them poor candidates to donate their organs. Hepatitis B is prevalent among the street dwellers of our metropolitan cities. Surveys have revealed that 7–10% of donors have this problem. There may be greater hazards. Medical reports from the Middle East speak of patients having contracted HIV infection from kidneys transplanted into them in Bombay.

These destitute individuals are easily recruited by the enterprising brokers. To a poor man on the streets, five thousand rupees is wealth beyond his wildest dreams. He is often unaware that the sum paid for his kidney is ten times that amount, and that the broker is taking the lion's share. Even if he discovers this, there is not much he can do about it. The broker has the resources and the organization to put him down. Most of the unrelated kidney transplants done in the country today are performed through these traders. Many of the transplant teams accept their services as a necessary evil, and excuse themselves by talking of the good they do to their suffering patients. There is, however, no way to conceal the fact that this is a trade in human organs.

Who are the sellers? No one who is comfortably off will undergo surgery, lose time from his work and suffer pain for someone he does not know. It is always the poor who sell their organs. We know that in the vast majority of cases the loss of a kidney does no harm. However, we also know that a donor can die as a direct result of the operation, either immediately from surgical complications, or later if he himself develops renal disease. I am aware of five donors who lost their lives in this way. We do not publish or publicize such failures, and it is unlikely that the donor will know about the risk, or that the knowledge will deter him in his desperate plight.

Newspapers carry horror stories of problems other donors face and of people being held incommunicado until the operation has taken place so that they will not change their minds. Worse still is the story that a young man went into hospital expecting to undergo surgery for a peptic ulcer and woke up minus a kidney. I do not believe all that appears in the press. Many stories may be concocted by young men trying to get some publicity, and eager reporters who know that sensational stories sell newspapers. However, I deplore the fact that these stories have enough credibility to find their place in print, and they do harm to legitimate transplant programs because people feel no transplantation related activity can be above suspicion.

Does the donor benefit in the long run? Unfortunately, no. Unused to having so much money, and being quite untrained in husbanding his resources, he ends up wasting the windfall on unproductive schemes, or lending it to the scores of relations and friends who immediately throng to share his good fortune, and within months he is back penniless on the pavement from which he came.

It is possible for the medical team to see that justice is done to the donor. There are some examples of doctors and hospitals who have supervised the whole transaction, who have made sure that the money is paid to the donor by a bank draft redeemable only in his home town, and that a health insurance policy is taken in his name. What more can they do? They cannot provide financial advice in the management of resources. They cannot ensure that the broker will not recover his pound of flesh later. All they have achieved is to take over the role of the broker to some extent. Is this the purpose of the medical profession?

Who are the beneficiaries of this scheme? Renal transplantation is a costly process. Fortunately, partial funding from Governments and service insurance programs have brought it within reach of the middle class, though not without difficulty. The added cost of buying a kidney and the need to use cyclosporin to achieve a reasonable chance of success makes unrelated live donor transplantation twice as costly as live related donor transplants. Only the very rich can afford unrelated donor transplantation, and only the very poor donate their kidneys. The very idea goes against all the principles of social justice. This is a classical case of the exploitation of the poor by the opulent. Should the medical profession be a party to this?

Bombay and Madras are the major centres of the kidney industry. The accessibility of these two cities to our wealthy neighbours from the Middle East and from Malaysia and Singapore has made it an export trade. Our poor are being exploited, not only by the upper classes of India, but also by the money bags of our neighbours.

What is the need for such programs? Those who run them always speak of their duty to their patients. How can they leave them in the lurch? The lack of transplantation does not kill those who can stay on dialysis. Today, high flux dialyzers have shortened dialysis times and improved well-being, and the availability of erythropoietin means that a patient on dialysis can be just as well as the one who has had a transplant. The only hitch is the high cost of dialysis. With the reuse procedures practised in our dialysis programs it is possible for a patient to mantain dialysis at home for a cost of Rs 2500/- a month. Against this is the cost of cyclosporin at Rs. 3000/- for five grams (not even a month's supply for a 60 kg Indian). A standard model artificial kidney costs no more than the transplant, and second hand machines are available for less. By stopping unrelated donor transplants, we will not be condemning our patients to death. They still have a very good prospect of healthy life on dialysis.

I must admit the force of two arguments in favour of the unrelated donor program. Since cyclosporin became available, the success rate of renal transplantation has improved and is now almost as good as that from related donors. Secondly, at debates held all over the country, it has become clear that the majority of the medical profession and the public are in favour of continuing with unrelated donor programs. I do not recognize the right of any external body or individual to interfere in what is an internal matter. It is for us as Indians to sort out this problem among ourselves.

One of the greatest objections I see to unrelated live donor transplantation is that it works against the establishment of cadaver organ donation. Indians are a conservative people, slow to change established traditions. A survey of public attitudes to cadaver organ donation carried out by the Tata Institute of Social Sciences in Bombay in 1980 revealed that only the well educated and the well informed were ready to donate their organs after death. In my own efforts to perform cadaver transplants in India, I have found that the few who were willing to donate the organs of their dead relations (approximately ten at the Jaslok Hospital between 1974 and 1983) were either relations of doctors or of patients. This is too small a minority to have any hope of establishing a program which could cover the needs of the country.

A feature of Indians in general is that we are easily influenced by example, and that we tend to accept some prominent people as leaders and to follow their precepts. The cadaver program therefore needs the weight of influence of consequential people in society for its success. Should one of them have renal failure today, what is likely to happen? It is unlikely that he will wish to accept the kidney of a member of his family, or that his relations would like to donate their organs. Today, it is easy for them to throw their money to a poor man and buy a kidney. If this were not possible, this influential body of men would be pressurizing Government and the public to organize cadaver transplant programs, and politicians would be likely to listen to them.

One special form of unrelated live donor program has been advocated, that of the emotionally related donor, usually the spouse. I am wary of accepting this in a country where marriages are still usually arranged. While most of us are enlightened, it is unfortunately true that brides are sometimes ill-treated to coerce their parents to provide a larger dowry. It would be too easy for a young man to marry for a kidney. Once married, no Indian woman will refuse to sacrifice anything for her husband.

It is obviously not going to be easy to break the practice of unrelated donor transplantation without providing a practical alternative. There is a pressing need for legislation to be introduced covering all forms of transplantation, not just the unrelated donor. There are malpractices today in the performance of live related donor transplants too. We need comprehensive legislation which would:

1. *Make it legal to remove organs for transplantation from adults after informed consent.* Nothing in Indian law today specifically permits this, and therefore the transplant team is always at risk of being accused of committing grievous hurt.
2. *Lay down criteria for the recognition of hospitals where such transplants may be done.* Too many transplants are being done in little nursing homes where there are no facilities to dialyze patients in whom transplants do not work, or to investigate reasons for failure. It is true that these institutions thrive because the recognized hospitals do not undertake unrelated donor transplants, and will be unable to draw patients if unrelated donor transplantation is not done.
3. *Prohibit the payment of any financial consideration to the donor of an organ transplant, whether related or unrelated.* It will be next to impossible to ensure this, but it may serve as a deterrent to the broker, who will be under suspicion.
4. *Stipulate that live donor transplantation may be done only if donor and recipient are at least haplo-identical.* This will eliminate the possibility of the medical team being deceived by the patient and the recipient, and being told they are related when they actually are not.
5. *Provide for cadaver organ transplantation by an opting out system, by which it may be assumed that every person is willing to donate his or her organs after death unless he or she has expressed unwillingness to do so.* Additionally, an opting in system may also be introduced, so that those who are very strongly motivated to donate their organs may specifically express that desire, and may carry an authorized donor card. This will help to persuade reluctant relatives to accept the wishes of the deceased at the time of death.
6. *Introduce criteria of brain death which can be applied in most hospitals in the country, and which do not call for much instrumentation.* The National Academy of Medical Sciences has already prepared and circulated a set of criteria for discussion among members of the profession.

There is some hope now that our State Governments are beginning to take action. (This is a State subject, according to the Indian Constitution.) After much lobbying by the National Kidney Foundation (India), the Government of Maharashtra passed a kidney transplant act in 1982. Unfortunately, they then went to sleep over the passing of rules which would make the act effective, but there is some sign of activity on that scene. The Government of Karnataka passed a similar act around 1987, and Tamil Nadu also followed suit in that year. The Tamil Nadu act was quite unworkable, as it called for the presence in the operating theatre of an officer of the Police Department not below the rank of a Sub-Inspector, hardly the easiest thing to organize in an emergency.

The solution to unrelated donor transplantation is an active cadaver transplant program and there is hope that we will see it in action soon.

Table 1. Unrelated live donor transplant programs. The arguments

For	Against
1. The patient without a related donor has no alternative but to take an unrelated kidney or to die.	1. Dialysis offers an effective means of treatment with good quality of life and is no more expensive.
2. The donor is a poor man who benefits from the money he earns by the sale of his kidney.	2. The donor rarely knows how to manage the wealth, and is soon back in extreme poverty.
3. It is possible to eliminate the middle man from the transaction and to safeguard the interests of the donor.	3. The middle man can be eliminated only if the doctor takes over his role, and is extremely vigilant.
4. Any risk to the donor of an unrelated kidney transplant is experienced equally by the related donor.	4. The related donor takes the risk out of love, and not out of financial necessity.
	5. Only the rich benefit. The poor lose their kidneys and risk their lives.
	6. Unrelated live programs will discourage cadaver transplantation.

14. Ethical problems in dialysis and transplantation: Africa

RASHAD S. BARSOUM

Abbreviations: RRT – Renal Replacement Therapy; ESRD – End-stage Renal Disease

I. Introduction

In Africa, the story dates back to around the middle of this century when the winds of Independence blew over the continent. They provoked an overwhelming sense of freedom and nationalism, together with enormous motivation to catch up with Western achievements. Yet the pace was too fast. It was both undesirable and impossible to avoid the progressive increase in the demands of people who were well aware of contemporary developments in the industrialized world. For an intellectual African to acquire the luxury accessible to the average American became a question of individual rights as well as national pride. It is very unfortunate that productivity, on the other hand, remained lagging far behind those dreams. Over the years, the balance between ambition and ability became totally disrupted, inflicting all the frustration that we see today.

One of the main areas in which both moral and material conflicts were expressed is health care. Driven by totally disorganized enthusiasm, nations possessing the necessary intellectual background continued to chase and import all possible kinds of advances in medical science and technology. It was realized too late that application was started before adopting any strategy, and that *practice* was started before *attitude*.

In this chapter, I shall try to analyze the ethical, moral and socio-economical consequences which emerged in several African communities. To give an outsider a clearer picture of the true situation, I shall start by giving some statistical data about renal disease and its management in Africa, then I shall try to analyze the attitudes of the four partners involved in the panorama, namely the patients, the public, the States and the physicians.

II. Renal disease in Africa

A. *Incidence*

Unfortunately, there are no reliable statistics on the incidence of renal disease in all African countries. However, there is a general impression that such diseases are

C. M. Kjellstrand and J. B. Dossetor (eds): Ethical Problems in Dialysis and Transplantation, 169–182.
© 1992 *Kluwer Academic Publishers. Printed in the Netherlands.*

170

very common, at least 3–4 times more common than they are in more developed countries. This is substantiated by analysis of the causes of death reported to the Health Authorities before the dialysis era, which suggests that uremia accounts for 1–1.5% of the total annual deaths among Egyptians, a figure which has remained steady for at least two decades [1]. This Figure is quite comparable to those obtained from other countries with similar socio-economic standards [2, 3, 4]. By further simple calculations, death from renal disease must be in the range of 200 per million of the general population.

There is also a general feeling that the incidence of renal disease is increasing, although there is yet no statistical evidence of this. Increasing public awareness is probably the major factor contributing to this impression. In addition, the outstanding moral, social and financial impact of the modern management of uremia seems to be falsely magnifying the size of renal disease as a health problem.

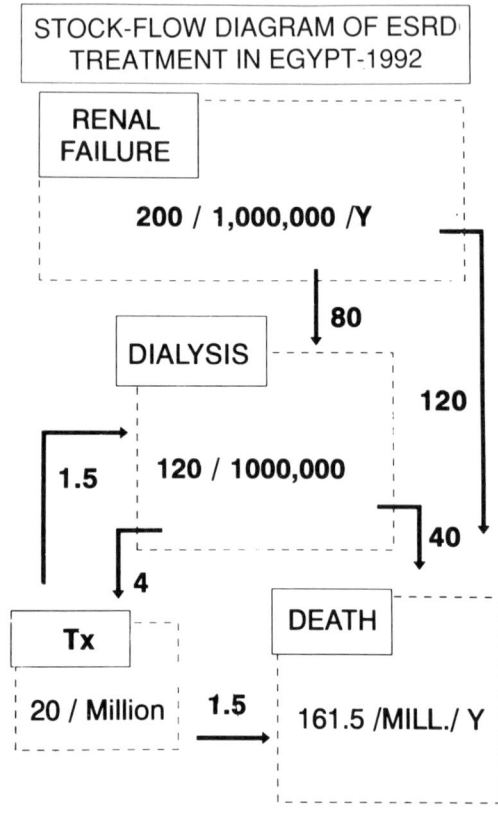

Figure 1. Stock-flow diagram of renal replacement therapy in Egypt, 1992. Numbers in dotted squares represent 'stocks'; general population of 50 millions, dialysis population of 6000 and transplant population of 1000 patients. Figures beside the arrows represent 'flow' of patients along different 'stocks' expressed per million of the general population.

Nevertheless, a true increase in the absolute number of renal failure patients is inevitable along with expansion in the size of population on renal replacement therapy (RRT). With the poor overall patient survival, this factor leads to an annual increase in dialysis population of some 15% (Figure 1). An added increment is associated with annual growth of the general population, which varies in different African countries from 2–7% [5].

Etiology

It is interesting that the calculated high incidence of End Stage Renal Disease (ESRD) in Africa is strikingly comparable with that of the black population in the United States [6]. However, the African figure is based on the Egyptian population, which is genetically a mixture of Caucasian, Negroid and Oriental [7]. It remains to be seen whether similar figures are obtained in back Africa, before making conclusions about the role of genetic factors.

In contrast to American blacks, Africans are exposed to an unique spectrum of nephritogenic environmental factors that undoubtedly reflect on the prevalence of renal disorders. Of these disorders, endemic infections are the most prominent. In most areas, man has learned how to survive with a tremendous load of parasitic [8], bacterial and viral infections [9]. Yet, beside other sequelae, the kidneys suffer considerable damage, directly or indirectly attributed to such agents. Thus, *schistosomiasis* is clearly responsible for lower urinary lesions leading to obstruction, reflux and ascending infection in millions of patients all over the continent [10]. In addition, the parasite provokes several immune reactions which end up with certain types of progressive *glomerulonephritis* and even *amyloidosis* [11]. Quartan malaria, mainly prevalent in Black Africa, still ranks as the commonest known cause of secondary nephrotic syndrome [12]. Membranous, and to a lesser extent, proliferative *glomerulonephritis*, are the main lesions atrributed to Plasmodium infection. Other parasitic diseases known to induce renal lesions with uncertain clinical significance include *Leishmaniasis* [13] found mainly in the East, *Ecchynococcosis* in the East and Northwest [14] and *Trypanosomiasis* in the Sub-Saharan regions of the continent [15] (Figure 2).

The epidemiological impact of these infestations on the prevalence of renal disease is difficult to measure. Rough estimates suggest that in at least 1/3 of patients with ESRD, renal disease may be atrributed to a previous parasitic infection [16].

Bacterial infections are also blamed. Streptococcal infections of the upper respiratory tract (consequent upon overcrowding in homes and schools) and the skin (complicating scabies) are still contributing to a high record of post-infectious *glomerulonephritis*. Chronic salmonellosis (frequently complicating *schistosomiasis*) is associated with distinct glomerular and interstitial lesions. Tuberculosis still ranks among the main causes of amyloidosis in Africa, let alone the direct renal damage induced by the mycobacterium.

Among the main viral infections, Hepatitis B seems to have an important

172

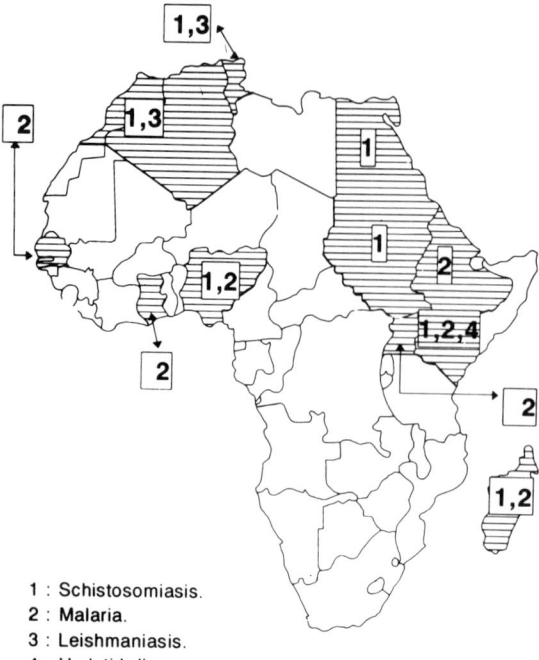

1 : Schistosomiasis.
2 : Malaria.
3 : Leishmaniasis.
4 : Hydatid disease.

Figure 2. Reported parasitic nephropathies in Africa.

bearing on the prevalence of steroid-resistant nephrotic syndrome among children in Southern and Western Africa [17]. The main renal lesion is membranous nephropathy, though the glomerular response in adults tends to be more proliferative. The epidemiologic impact of other endemic viral infections, such as CMV, HBV and HIV on the prevalence of renal disease, so far, seems negligible.

Attention has been recently focused on the potential role of the African abiotic environment in inducing renal disease. Environmental pollution composed of endless natural and man-made ingredients is overwhelming. On the basis of animal experiments, almost everything from artificial sweeteners to packing material, the use of which is absolutely out of any State control, can cause considerable interstitial renal injury. Of these thousand of potentially harmful chemicals, heavy metals seem to constitute an imminent threat. The most eligible candidate is lead, being an abundant impurity in low quality motor car fuel and some alcoholic drinks. The effect of this substance bypasses the frame of occupational exposure, amounting to the level of general environmental pollution in large and overcrowded African cities. Studies are under way to see whether or not lead and other environmental impurities are responsible for the extremely high incidence of *idiopathic* interstitial nephropathy in many African countries.

III. Management

At the point where an African patient becomes uremic, it all depends on his *power*, whether or not he will eventually receive adequate management. The rich, the *star* and the influential can receive first class treatment, usually available in the private sector, in the same or neighbouring city or country. This applies to all modern therapeutic modalities including hospital, satellite and home hemodialysis, IPD, CAPD, and live-donor transplantation. The *ordinary* patient who cannot afford anything other than subsidized treatment has to suffer to a greater or lesser extent, depending on the country where he lives.

Owing to the different situation in South Africa, I shall exclude its highly developed system of RRT from this discussion. Large dialysis programs are available in the five Northern African countries bordering the Mediterranean, namely Egypt, Libya, Tunisia, Algeria and Morocco. By far the largest is the Egyptian, with about 6,000 patients receiving treatment in over 100 dialysis units (of which about 1/3 are private). This represents 12 per million of the general population, and as depicted in Figure 1, accommodates 80 new patients per million per year, estimated as 40% of those actually needing dialysis [9]. Selection is theoretically made on the first-come/first-serve principle, but in actual fact, many potential candidates never show up, being lost somewhere at the level of the general practictioner, poorly informed specialist, or most usually, transfer bureaucracy. The State *sponsors* dialysis treatment by a nominal reimbursement that is considered enough to cover all the direct expenses of State-owned units. This payment, however, covers about 70% of the actual expenses as calculated in market oriented private units. Patients have to pay the difference if they choose the private sector.

With a few exceptions, there is a remarkable difference in the results of treatment in terms of mortality, morbidity and rehabilitation, between State- and private- units. Although, part of this difference may be related to the socio-economic and educational standards of patients, there is however an undoubted financial influence that affects the quality of service and staff motivation.

There are several successful transplant programs of which about 50% are sponsored and run by the State, that also subsidizes some 30–50% of the expenses in private hospitals. The total annual capacity of these programs is about 400 cases, all from living donors. The ethical values differ among various centers; some accept only related donors, others accept spouses and emotionally-related donors, and still others do not mind *financially-motivated* donors. The State does not interfere, though it has recently illegalized donations from Egyptians to foreigners in an attempt to abort a growing market. Since money is very commonly involved irrespective of the type of donor, transplantation is more readily available to those who can financially afford it. The results favourably compare with international standards but with a higher patient mortality, due to the understandably higher incidence of opportunistic infections.

Renal dialysis services in the Northwest countries, Morocco, Algeria, and Tunisia [18] are widely spread and very well developed, covering an average of some 12 patient per million population [19]. The State's contribution is extensive, though there is still some place for a growing private activity. Modest local transplant programs are developing, but so far have been restricted to live-related donors. Yet the majority of transplants, largely from cadaver donors, are still done in France at an extremely high cost, also covered by the State.

Libya has only recently joined the club, with two state-owned and run foci. These are providing nephrology and dialysis services to the whole country – but with a very busy schedule that can only accommodate a minority of patients with ESRD. Many transplants are done in neighbouring countries, mainly Egypt, Kuwait and India, but local live-related transplant programs were started about a couple of years ago, with the help of visiting teams.

The only other African country with comparable standards is Kenya, though most activity, which includes dialysis and live-related transplantation is owned by the private sector and restricted to the capital, Nairobi. There is virtually no chronic RRT in the rest of the continent [20]. In some countries such as Sudan, Ethiopia, Tanzania and Madagascar in the East, and Nigeria in the West, facilities are modest and available mostly for acute dialysis. Little room is left for patients with chronic renal failure who come for treatment sporadically. Occasional live-related donor transplants have been done over the past two decades in Sudan but most transplants are currently done in neighbouring countries, usually Egypt. This, of course, is available only to the rich.

In the remaining African countries even acute hemodialysis may not be available. Chronic renal failure patients are simply left to die unless they can manage to move abroad for transplantation.

IV. Partners involved in the panorama

For proper appraisal of the impact of uremia therapy in Africa, I have chosen to highlight the attitudes of each of the principal four components of the scene, mainly ESRD patients, the Public, State health authorities and the medical profession.

A. *The African uremic patient*

Once declared to be uremic, the African patient starts a long, tough struggle for survival, during which he is bound to face unnumerable difficulties, threats and disappointments. Most patients are frustrated by the discrepancy between how much they expect and how much they get of medical and social support.

Their expectations on one hand, largely depend on their knowledge about the modern treatments of ESRD and their applicability in the industrialized world. This, in turn, depends on the individual patient's cultural and educational level as well as on the standard of public information available. Both factors vary from one African community to another, reflecting the prevailing life style, which is influenced by cultural, economical and political standards. The painful fact is that all factors selectively work against the publicity of treatment among the poor and uneducated. Though admittedly unfair, this mercifuly diminishes their frustration.

On the other hand, the relative shortage of facilities in practically all African communities inevitably imposes the concept of patient selection. This must bring back to Western communities the painful memories of Selection Boards of the sixties, that had to decide who was to live and who was to die. Whatever might be said about the inherent injustice in such Board decisions, they were undoubtedly much more fair and predictable when compared with the selection procedures currently supervening in the Third World.

Here, it is *power* that dictates. Rich patients readily find their way into the better-equipped private dialysis units where they have better chances of survival and rehabilitation. They can eventually afford rewarding a poor *emotionally-related friend* for donating a kidney for transplantation. So, in effect, the rich can simply *buy* a better life.

Power is not only money. Politicians, high rank civil servants and public opinion leaders have enough power to open many closed doors. They have a much better chance of being selected for State-sponsored dialysis and transplantation. It is shameful to admit that even within the same centre such patients usually receive special care that reflects positively on the results of their treatment.

This is the sad picture of the selection process, prevailing in practically all African and other Third World countries. It can then be understood how bitter the ordinary patient must feel in this atmosphere of injustice, which explains the whole spectrum of reactions that vary from depression to aggression.

B. *ESRD and the African public*

A trip along African countries may be taken as an adventure by the legendary Time Machine. Despite all the differences in culture, economy and politics, African cultures can be linked, as far as the management of uremia is concerned, in one evolutionary scale.

At the far distant end in tribal communities of Central Africa, there is no problem [1]. No treatment is available for chronic renal failure, but the public is unaware of any shortage. Many patients are misdiagnosed, and the question of long-term dialysis is not raised anyway.

In more advanced communities, usually those living in the big African cities, people are generally aware of the disease and its treatment modalities but they do not bother to think about it. Involved families, however, are bound to suffer from the direct social and financial consequences of having to live with a partially disabled patient, spouse or son on regular dialysis.

Further forward in the scale are communities where renal transplantation is available. In virtually all African countries this practice is precocious. It is invariably started by a few ambitious and competent medical groups who are able to realize the dream by performing a few successful live-related donor transplants. The spark spreads among thousand of dialysis patients who start looking around for the idealistic *generous relative* willing to donate a kidney. Although this may work, many disappointments occur, leading to eventual disruption of seemingly excellent family ties. Sometimes, even if the *good* brother is located and all social barriers overcome, some form of reward is expected. This does not need to be money. A precious gift, an expensive flat, a small car or a free share in business may do. I have seen established wills being changed as a part of such deals.

More liberal communities in the capitals further rationalize paid organ donation. Since some form of material benefit is, anyway, accepted *'dans la famille'*, why couldn't this concept be stretched a little to involve distant relatives and friends as well? Why should not this even involve any suitable and willing citizen who is after all a brother in the big family, community, country?! Compromization continues under the pressure of an increasing number of patients who are ready to pay in the face of progressive general socio-economic deterioration. The unemployed ambitious young man earning less that $300 a year must seriously consider an offer of $10,000 if he is to donate a kidney to save the life of a dialysis-dependant beautiful young lady who could very well be his sister. The doctors assure him that the operation is safe with virtually no future ill consequences; all that he may suffer is a little post-operative pain and a couple of weeks in hospital. Covered with the blessings of his community the young man finds it only logical to accept the deal. He would even regard himself as a coward if he does not.

Selling kidneys has always been rationalized by good-will, the desperate need for money being the common dominator. The father who cannot feed his children, the wife who has literally no hope of surviving if her spouse and only sponsor needs an expensive and life-saving surgery, the brother who has no means to support his only sister's marriage are true and common models depicting the nobel motives that justify the selling of organs. A community that cannot, in the first place, avoid the existence of such desperate situations, has no choice but to praise the heroes who are able to change their life-styles by brave decisions.

Having gained acceptance of the public opinion, paid organ donation finds good soil wherever the rich are too rich and the poor are too poor. Very soon, the noble motives behind donation are forgotten and only the material part of the deal remains. Professional donors develop, far from being devoted, sacrificing and brave. Their only motive is to gain easy money which they do not even have any plans to spend. Some do not even have any intention to donate; they just *blackmail* their potential recipients during the initial phases of medical assessment, only to quit shortly before the final steps. Playing this game with two or more recipients per year can make up for their living. The passive community, preoccupied by major public and individual problems closes its eyes hoping not to see this corruption. Nevertheless, a religious leader or a new political figure emerges from time to time, exposing the dirty side of paid organ donation for different reasons that are not always genuine. Conferences are held, hot speeches delivered and strong statements made to condemn paid organ donation. But the storm eventually cools down, and the selling of organs continues and expands to become one of the facts of life in poor communities with precocious transplant activities.

C. *The African health authorities*

African governments are overwhelmed by enormous problems. Health care as a whole is only one of such problems and does not even score high enough in the scale of priorities. Prevention of disease, which should be the principal target, is largely handicapped by illiteracy, poverty and poor hygiene. Besides, prevention programs are, after all, long-term investment projects with no visible immediate revenue, a fact that politically aborts many sincere attempts. For these reasons and others, endemic diseases continue to flourish with innumerable consequences.

Primary health care suffers equal shortcomings. Even such simple health problems as perinatal mortality, infantile diarrhea and other infectious diseases continue to kill millions of children in underdeveloped countries.

Secondary care, on the other hand, is the main facade of health care in developing countries. To the layman, the politician and the opinion leader, it is the synonym of *health care* as a whole. In countries where politics have such an impact on public services as they do in Africa, it is no wonder that secondary care consumes most of the health budget.

It was in this atmosphere, where a critical balance was hardly established between health requirements, public pressures, politics and finance, that the issue of tertiary care emerged. It is certainly both the duty of health authorities and their pride to support the application of high technology in medicine. There is also no doubt that adoption of sophisticated medical care in a particular hospital improves the standard of all related disciplines. But what is the price? How can it be acceptable to spend the whole average annual income of ten citizens in order to provide dialysis treatment for one uremic? How can we rationalize spending all that is needed to feed thirty infants in order to cover one transplant for one year?

In most African countries, there are no current possibilities of any significant financial support by the public for the adoption of medical high technology. Although some insurance schemes are present in the Northern Countries, many others are lagging behind. There are no private enterprises of such a size that can even fully cover their own staff. Donations are largely restricted by the overall poor financial standards and political insecurity.

Eventually it is the overloaded government that, despite all constraints, has to cover the expenses of tertiary health care for practically all patients, save the very few who choose not to request State support. Since State hospitals cannot cover all the demands, governments in most African countries have developed partial reimbursement schemes for private RRT.

Although this policy has created a healthy competition between private centers, the lack of careful quality control has encouraged many centers to compromise with quality for price. This, among other factors, is certainly responsible for the strikingly high morbidity and mortality encountered in such units.

D. *Medical profession*

Expectations of the renal physician in Africa exceed those from his colleagues in the West by far. This may be the legacy of a long heritage from epochs when the physician was a philosopher, a priest or a magician according to culture. It also stems from almost legendary biographies of Western missionaries and volunteers serving in the continent at the turn of the century, who actually established the basis of modern medical and nursing practice. Their influence was not technical in as much as it was moral, turning their image into that of *leaders* rather than *doctors*. Contemporary physicians are not by essence of the same caliber. Although they continue to be among the most educated, cultured and sophisticated, they are not necessarily philosophers, magicians or missionaries!

Today's average physician regards the scope of clinical practice as largely confined to the arts and techniques of diagnosis and the skills and rules of management. He is usually unqualified for, disinterested in, and indeed bored from being involved in the social, political and financial issues always emerging in the context of patient care. This attitude, the justification of which is questionable, obviously fails the expectations of all other partners involved in the dilemma of modern ESRD therapy.

Most patients are disappointed. They usually cannot see the point in any selection system adopted by any medical team, that eventually classifies them under different priorities. The bitterness of the poor when they realize that the rich enjoy the priority of private treatment, is all poured on the faces of their physicians. Even the few who are lucky to be accepted in a State-sponsored program are disappointed by the relatively modest technical and staffing standards. Failure of an expanding pool of dialysis patients to find suitable donors for transplantation creates a growing criticism against physicians who should have been much more active in establishing kidney banks.

Public opinion is generally hostile against renal physicians. After all the taxes which have been collected, all the wages paid to physicians, nurses, technicians and bioengineers, all the incredible fees which private doctors charge and all those conferences, symposia and debates, the medical profession has not only failed to treat patients well, but also exported to the community those innumerable, social, moral, ethical and financial problems involved in the management of ESRD. Physicians keep on asking for more funds, donations and equipment. They want to change the law hoping to have the rights of playing with the bodies of the dead even without consent. They are pushing society to cast aside a long heritage of respecting the bodies of the dead, traditionally expressed by their burial intact. They have even encouraged the development of a kidney marketing business aiming only at financial gains or, at least, personal pride. They have simply gone too far.

Governments are even more disappointed. Nephrologists seem to have totally distracted themselves from the scope of public health services. How can they claim priority for a disease that accounts for only 1–2% of the annual mortalities? How can they embarrass the health authorities by developing and publicizing such expensive treatments which create an expanding pool of at least partially disabled, highly demanding people? Where are their efforts to reduce cost or to find cheaper solutions? How did they have the guts to accept paid organ donations that created all that chaos in the community and threw a terrible financial burden on the State?

It is true, in my opinion, that the medical profession has been rather passive in reacting to this whole dilemma. Only a minority of physicians in different countries realize the importance of the socio-economic and political dimensions in treating uremic patients. Getting involved in such issues needs knowledge, time, courage and nerves. For an honest and moral stand, one has to face and compromise with all partners involved. No one physician can do it alone, hence the importance of medical associations. Nephrological societies, of which there are less than a dozen in the whole African continent, have subsequently acquired socio-political trends in addition to their scientific duties.

Nevertheless, there are considerable strategic disagreements about several critical issues within such professional societies. For example, there is no clear resolution as to whether an organized patient-selection system for RRT should be adopted. Some physicians have the feeling that it is their duty, as nephrologists, to defend the rights of all uremic patients to be treated irrespective of available funds. In their opinion, the Society should negotiate on their behalf with health authorities for higher budgets, should encourage donations, and indeed knock at every door of potential funding source. Others are convinced that public health is a general issue in which priorities must be respected. Any available funds, from whatever source they are derived, must be entered into the pool of health services and spent according to those priorities. This necessitates setting clear-cut parameters for defining priorities as well as a patient selection system.

In the face of such disagreement on the essence of physicians' attitudes towards renal replacement therapy, patients established their own associations, the membership of which also includes sympathetic nephrologists. There obviously support the unselective policy and consider themselves as the only body qualified to speak for the principal consumer of RRT services, namely, the patient. Nevertheless, African renal patient associations have not acquired enough political independence, and most of them are still working under the umbrella of medical societies.

Most African Nephrological Societies are trying to bridge the gap between patient requirements and demands on one hand and the official and public's responses on the other. The Egyptian Society of Nephrology, as an example, took over the task of setting the standards of proper dialysis services, estimating the realistic cost and establishing a reliable registry. Dialysis units that comply are acknowledged by the society, this so far being a prestigious advantage. Although health authorities encourage these initiatives, they do not force the society recommendations into action, nor do they even apply them in State-sponsored units. It is hoped that while negotiations continue, the superiority of society-acknowledged units will leave no place for any further State reluctance.

The same Society is currently leading a campaign to support cadaver organ transplantation as the only foreseeable exit from the current economical, moral and professional chaos. Through innumerable symposia, lectures, workshops and even private talks, members of the Society are trying to create a moral consensus of opinion and to impose the necessary legislations which will permit the harvesting of organs from heart-beating cadavers. Similar efforts have been successful in the Northwest African countries, yet are still lagging behind in all others.

Through personal acquaintances and public relations, nephrologists are also trying to raise independent funds for the support of RRT programs. Such attempts have been successful in opening a few dialysis units and sponsoring a few transplant hospital beds. Yet the magnitude of such contributions is still too limited to be taken into account in budget planning, and too sporadic to initiate a general feeling of true interaction between uremic patients and their communities.

V. The Utopia of RRT treatment

The question remains, is there any hope of providing *decent* care for *all* African ESRD patients, without having to pay all this price of frustration and corruption? My answer is *yes*.

In the first place, it is vital to have precise information about the components of the well-acknowledged stock-flow formula of renal patients in every country.

The dialysis pool should be rigid, as small as possible, and proportionate to a prospectively allocated realistic fund which should be enough to provide an optimal technical standard. By contrast, the transplant pool should be expansile, largely based on cadaver donor donation, though a few live-related donor transplants with excellent matching may be included for obvious reasons.

Accommodating the whole potential input, which will be comprised of all new patients as well as returns from the transplant pool, has to be the final goal. Until this is achieved, a clear-cut and highly respected selection policy must be adopted. The criteria of selection will vary in different countries, but all efforts must be made to decrease the time on dialysis and increase availability of transplantation. This is basically achievable by having a wide access to cadaver organ transplantation. This is an area that needs a lot of work including legislation, public opinion orientation, funding, promotion of causality and intensive care services, development of numerous efficient harvesting and transplanting teams and allocation of enough, optimally equipped hospitals and post-transplant follow-up clinics.

By a good system of organization, not only is the dialysis pool balance achievable, but also its transit time shortened. Dialysis would then be more cost-effective, long-term complications will be reduced, patient and staff morale improved and their interaction enhanced.

Stagnant lanes will undoubtedly developed in the dialysis pool, comprising patients who are unfit or unwilling to be transplanted as well as an inevitably growing population of pre-sensitized subjects mostly coming back from unsuccessful transplants. Unless the dialysis pool is allowed to expand, these lanes must have a negative effect on the flow and subsequently on the flexibility of selection criteria. Another factor that has a similar influence is the rapid population growth rate supervening in most African countries, that must extrapolate to the number of patients needing dialysis. Calculating the effects of these factors is essential for future projections, if the flow is to be kept most optimal.

For the establishment of this Utopia of RRT in Africa, all partners must sit together, ignore all personal factors and all previous conflicts, get rid of the famous third world priority bias, and work hard for a conceivable and achievable goal. Is this practically possible in Africa? This is the question.

References

1. Barsoum RS, Rihan ZEB, Ibrahim AS et al. Long-term intermittent hemodialysis in Egypt. Bull WHO 1974; 51: 647–54.
2. Abdulla K. Chronic renal failure in Northern Iraq. Iraqi Mid J 1979; 27: 43–6.
3. Friedman EA, Delano BG. Can the world afford uremia therapy? Proc 8th Int Congr Nephrol, Athens 1981; 57–83.
4. Abdullah MS. Development of renal services in Kenya. East Afr Med J 1981; 30: 9–10.
5. World Health Organisation. Annual Statistics Report 1988.
6. Gordon D. Racial differences in ESRD. Dial and Transplant 1990; 19: 114–6.
7. Kamel MA, Fouad MY, Mahfouz M et al. Population analysis of HLA-A and B genetic markers in 1000 Egyptians. Med J Cair Univ 1984; 52: 507–10.
8. Barsoum RS. Parasitic nephropathies. Medical Forum 1990; 35: 19–23.
9. Barsoum RS. Nephrology and African Ecology. Proc VII World Congress of ISAO, Sapporo, Japan; 1989.
10. Iarotski LC, Davis A. The schistosomiasis problem in the world: results of a WHO questionnaire survey. Bull WHO 1981; 59: 115–27.
11. Barsoum RS. Schistosomal glomerupathy: Selection factors. Nephrol Dial Transplant 1987; 2: 488–97.
12. Hendirekse RB, Aderriyi A. Quartan malarial nephrotic syndrome in children. Kidney Int 1979; 16: 64–74.
13. De Brito T, Hoshimo-Schimizu S, Amarto Neto V et al. Glomerular involvement in human Kala-azar. Am J Trop Med Hyg 1975; 1: 29–31.
14. Okelo GBA, Kyobe J. A three-year review of human hydatid disease seen at Kenyata National Hospital. East Afr Med J 1981; 58: 695–6.

182

15. Nagle RB, Ward PA, Lindsky HB *et al*. Experimental infections with African trypanosomiasis. Am J Trop Med Hyg 1974; 23: 15–18.16. El-Said W. Nephrology in Egypt. Proceedings of ISN African Kidney and Electrolytes Conference, Cairo Egypt. Center for Medical Education, Cairo University Press 1988; 196–200.
17. Seggie J, Nathoo K, Davies PG. Association of hepatitis B (HBs) antigenaemia and membranous glomerulo-nephritis in Zimbabwean children. Nephron 1984; 38: 115–119.
18. El-Matri A, Ben Maiz H, Ben Abdullah T *et al*. Traitment de l'insuffisance renale chronique en Tunisie. Proc 14e Congres Medicale Magh 1985.
19. Tufveson G, Geerlings W, Brunner FP *et al*. 1989: Combined report on regular dialysis and transplantation in Europe XIX, 1988. Proc Eur Dial Transplant Ass 1989; 4: 6–7.
20. Barsoum RS. Ethical and moral dilemmas arising from uremic therapy in the Third World – A 'KAP' Review. Prog in Artificial Organs 1985; 89–95.

15. Japanese view on life and organ transplantation

KAŻUHIKO ATSUMI

Japan is one of the advanced countries. Almost 95% of medical care in Japan is covered by the National Health Insurance and practised with high technology throughout the country. It is estimated that 200,000 ultrasonic echograms, 70,000 dialyzers, 20,000 X-Ray CT scanner, 2,000 MRI imaging systems, etc. are in use in Japan, a country with a population of 120 million.

However, a discrepancy can be seen in the area of clinical use of organ transplantation. Although corneal and renal transplantation have already been approved legally, the number of kidney transplantations done in Japan is very small in comparison with other countries such as the USA and Europe.

I. Japanese status of organ transplantation

As of 1987, the total number of kidney transplantations done in Japan numbered 5,328. During 1987 alone, 572 kidney transplantations were carried out. In comparison with the USA (8,967 in 1987), and Europe (9,216 in 1986), the Japanese number is quite small (Figure 1).

The proportion of related live donor kidneys used was 75.7% for 1984–1987 (79.4% for 1987). In comparison with USA (21.3% in 1987) and Europe (11.0% in 1986) it is clear that the Japanese related live donor porportion is much higher than for cadaveric kidneys. Most living kidney donors were parents (57%).

From January 1980 to February 1985 there were 105 cases of kidney transplantation from brain death donors. This is extremely small compared to the USA and Europe. The longest survival time of a kidney transplant recipient in Japan is 21 years.

On the other hand, the total number of dialysis patients was 80,553 in 1987 of whom of 96.9% were treated by hemodialysis and the other 3.1% by CAPD. The number of patients who have had ten years of dialysis is 12,094 and the longest survival time is 21 years and 4 months.

According to medical statistics, morbidity and death due to kidney disease in Japan is similar to those of other developed countries. However, a significant discrepancy can be seen in the method of treatment. In 1986, 3.3% of renal failure

183

C. M. Kjellstrand and J. B. Dossetor (eds): Ethical Problems in Dialysis and Transplantation, 183–188.
© 1992 *Kluwer Academic Publishers. Printed in the Netherlands.*

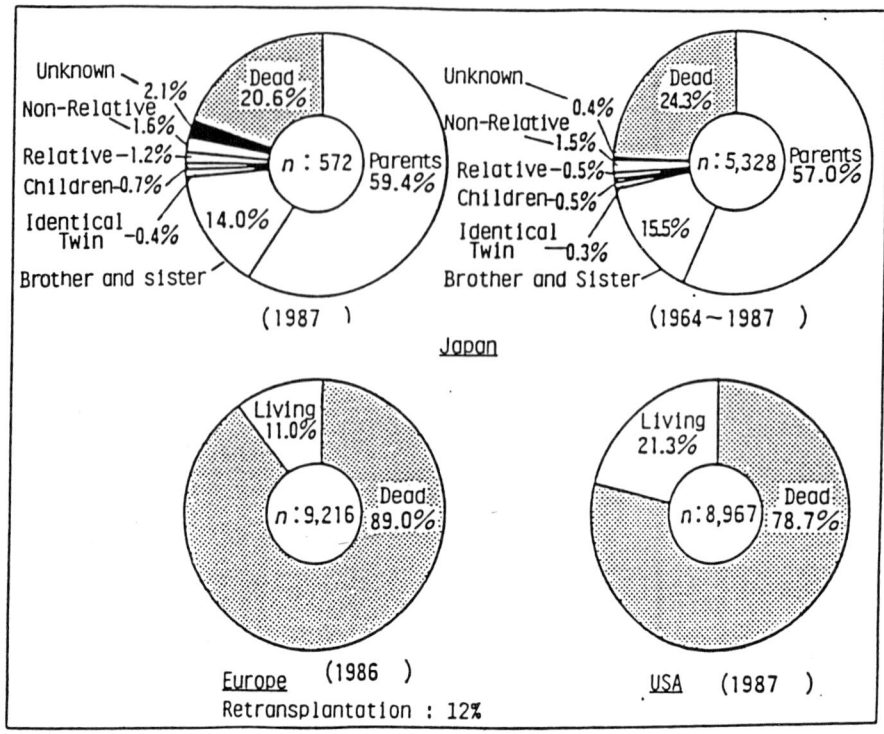

Figure 1. Classification of Donors in Kidney Transplantation in Japan, USA and Europe.

patients received kidney transplantation, with the remaining 96.7% were treated by dialysis (Figure 2). The ratio would be considered exceptionally out-of-balance for renal failure management in other developed countries.

In 1968 the first clinical case of heart transplantation was performed by Dr J. Wada. Since then no cardiac transplantation has been done in Japan, until recently. The first patient survived for three months but there were ethical problems in regard to confirmation of brain death in the donor.

Why is the clinical application of organ transplantation underdeveloped in Japan? Many reasons have been discussed for this deficiency, such as ethical problems with the first cardiac transplantation, Japanese traditional customs being against the practice of donating organs, Japanese life values reject the concept of brain death, a deficit of philanthropy in Japanese minds, or materialism in the younger generation, etc.

Recently, there have been many debates on the question of brain death for transplantation, not only in the medical profession but in the also mass media. In this respect, last year an advisory committee was organized by the ministry of Health and Welfare at the national level to discuss brain death.

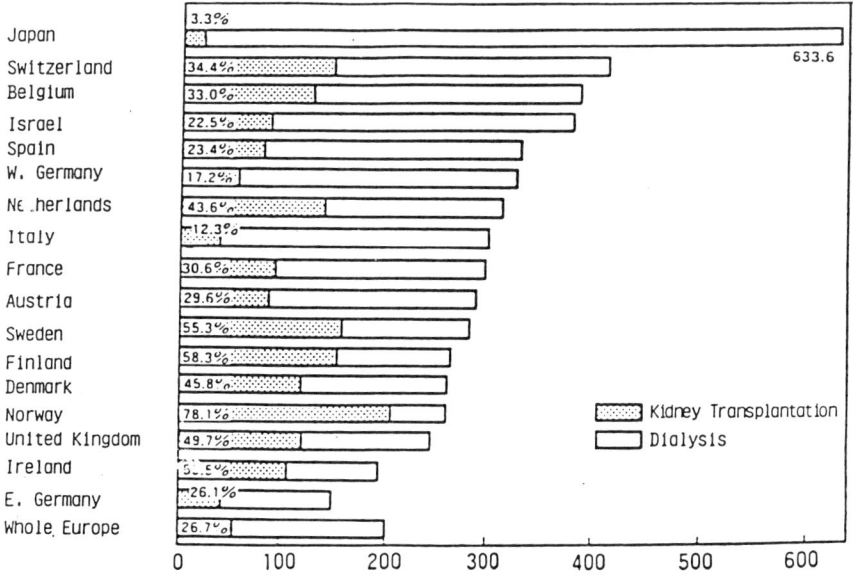

Figure 2. Comparison between Kidney Transplantation and Dialysis in Various Countries.

II. Questionnaire on brain death and organ transplantation

Many questionnaires on brain death have been carried out in Japan. Ten years ago, the ratio of acceptance by professionals of the theory that 'brain death is human death' was quite low (10–15%), however, the ratio has been increasing year by year, and last year's questionnaire showed a fairly high acceptance of 65%. On December 6, 1990, the Advisory Committee on Brain Death and Organ Transplantation reported on the topic of 'Is brain death recognized as human death?' According to the report, 731 out of 1,000 individuals responded, and the results are as follows:

Yes – Brain death is human death	66.3%
No – Brain death is not human death	16.3%
Did not Know	17.4%

The percentage of 'yes' responders in different categories of professionals was as follows: Medical related – 80.4%, Policy maker – 78.8%, Industry – 75.0%, Mass media – 72.4%, Religion related – 50.%, Legal related – 51.8%. The reasons most often given against the concept of brain death being recognized as human death were: 1) 'only heartbeat cessation is human death' – 42.9%, 2) MD's diagnosis of brain death cannot be accepted – 42.9%.

On December 15, 1990, NHK, The National Television Company, conducted an interesting questionnaire on brain death for medical professionals and non-professionals, asking the following questions:

1. 'Do you feel brain death was the cause of your relative's death?'

This question was given to families whose relatives were identified by medical professionals as having died from brain death. Non-professional responses ($n = 134$) were YES – 30%, NO – 70%.

2. 'Do you persuade the family to disconnect the respirator from the patient who is judged to be brain dead?'

Professionals (neurosurgeons and emergency care doctors) responded ($n = 100$): YES – 44%, NO – 56%.

3. 'Can you rely on the judgement of brain death by medical doctors?'

Non-professionals' responses: YES – 44%, NO – 22%, DO NOT KNOW – 34%.

4. 'Regarding confirmation of brain death, is there any defect in medical organizational structure?'

Professionals' responses: YES – 48%, NO – 52%.

5. 'Are there deficiencies in any of the following aspects of medical organizational structures?'

Professionals' affirmative responses, in percentages:

i) Relationship between doctors and patients	7%
ii) Doctors' protection of each other	6%
iii) Is of a small group of unqualified MDs?	43%
iv) Miscellaneous aspects	44%

The low acceptance and recognition of brain death may be mainly related to traditional Japanese social customs and cultural history, although some refusal to accept the concept relates to distrust of Japanese doctors.

Japanese doctors find it interesting that 61% of donors for organ transplantation in USA are white, 25% are Hispanic, 7% are Black, 2% are 'others', and only 1% are Japanese. In contrast, a recent questionnaire given to 100 medical doctors in Osaka University Hospital showed that 91% of medical doctors were willing to donate their organs in a brain death situation.

III. Japanese life values

More than 2000 years ago, as stated in the 'Kojiki', the famous historical book of Japan, the region of 'Yomi no kuni' or 'Meido' was described as a region where the dead could be found wandering under the tombs. According to the story the

Japanese god 'Izanagi no mikoto' visited the 'Yomi no kuni' where he met his dead lover, 'Izanami no mikoto'. He was so surprised to see her dirty and ruined body that he promptly fled from the 'Yomi no kuni', and put a huge stone against the opening to the region to protect himself from pursuit by her spirit. In the ancient Japanese mind, when facing death, there was no feeling that this was fate, and no belief in retribution for one's sins. Therefore, there was no hope for relief by salvation and no fear of punishment. The concept of retribution did not exist. In other words, 'Yomi no kuni' was recognized as having the property of purity or impurity, but not good or evil. It can be said that death had no ethical meaning, but was recognized as a physical phenomenon.

In Europe, because of the teaching of the apostle Paul, there was a decisive change in belief concerning the significance of death. Since then, people have been afraid that death is a time of penance for sin, in an ethical sense. In the ancient Hellenic world, the concept of retribution and judgement after death was deeply connected with the immortality of the soul (an essential aspect of Christianity).

As time passed, humans began to understand that justice cannot be achieved in the real world, and veered towards guarantees for the realization of justice after death. In order to permit this, immortality of the soul was considered to be indispensable.

On the other hand, the 'Jyodokyo', one of the edicts of Japanese Buddhism, had great impact in establishing Japanese values of life and death with the concept that salvation comes solely through the benevolence of Amitabha Buddha. In the beliefs of 'Jyodokyo', the next world is not the place to atone for sins, but the place to be compensated for injustice and evil. The mild illusions of 'Jyodokyo' may contribute to making the death of a Japanese more gay and less serious. 'Jyodokyo' teaches the unique esthetic that even punishment can be dispelled by the beautification of death. The ancient Japanese believe that 'death is impure' is now transformed to the Samurai's belief that 'death is pure.' In this way, the Samurai doctrine 'not to fear death' was generated and proceeded thereafter to inform Japanese traditional thinking.

IV. The characteristics of Japan

Japan consists of several islands and is isolated by other countries by the sea, therefore Japan has no experience of foreign invasion and few influences from foreign cultures. Japan is a small country, and populated by a single race speaking a single language. Consequently, the central region's culture can easily be transmitted to the periphery; there is cultural homogeneity.

From a geographical point of view, Japan lies in the temperate zone with lots of trees and flowers and the climate is mild and beautiful. In addition, seasonal changes are distinct all year round, from spring to winter. Consequently, Japanese are considered to be sensitive to subtle changes in surroundings and have a tendency to fuse with nature. Co-existence with nature is one of the traditional characteristics of the Japanese personality. The Japanese view of reality has been generated by this co-existence with nature.

V. Japanese rationalism

It used to be considered that Japanese culture was intuitive rather than rationalistic, and that duty and human feelings were dominant in Japanese thinking. However, as time has passed, this has changed. The value of duty – ie: the Chinese moral principle in 'Zukyo' – was introduced to Japan from China in the 12th century. The concept of reason in the 'Shushigaku' of Chinese philosophy, which is related to 'Zukyo' gave great impetus to Japanese rationalism. Rationalism is generally divided into two aspects, transcendent rationalism and empirical rationalism. In modern Japan empirical rationalism is the more acceptable concept.

Compatibility of reason with human feeling in empirical rationalism is deeply related to the Japanese view of nature. The Japanese view of reality cherishes the relationship of all material substances, though it is deficient in unifying them into a single whole system.

VI. Japanese views on transplantation

The Japanese attitude to organ transplantation is far behind the medical progress in the rest of the world, in spite of acceptance of other medical advances. According to some questionnaires, the reason hinges on Japanese distrust for the medical community and, in particular, the previously mentioned ethical problem with respect to the first heart transplant. However, other major causes for this deficiency derive from the Japanese view of life and its traditional culture and religion. Buddhism has been considered as one of the reasons that the Japanese did not accept organ transplantation, yet heart transplantations have been carried out in Thailand where Buddhism is strictly practised. 'Zukyo' was also considered to be one of the reasons as in this doctrine damage to organs is strongly prohibited, yet heart transplantations are performed in Taiwan where 'Zukyo' is one of the traditional principles of teaching.

The majority of Japanese believe in the immortality of the soul and the soul will remain with the body, even after death. This is why funeral events are so gorgeous in Japan in order to unburden the soul. It may seem peculiar to some that Japanese families try so hard to claim the bodies of relatives who have died in an airplane accident, even when this is supremely difficult. They will put forth a great effort to achieve this.

The Japanese view on brain death and organ transplantation will be changed in the future through steady education and scientific advances in the medical community. The concept of brain death is sure to be accepted in Japan by the next century, and citizens will benefit from transplant therapy.

16. A different view from different countries: Eastern Europe

I. Abstract

The development of renal replacement therapy (RRT) has not been uniform in all parts of the world. It was the most rapid in the United States of America and Japan, slower in Western Europe, slower yet in Eastern Europe and negligible in the developing countries of the Mediterranean. The rapid growth of dialysis and transplant activity in the West was caused by the availability of sophisticated dialysis technology and money. The number of End Stage Renal Disease (ESRD) patients on renal replacement therapy (RRT) is related to the gross national product (GNP) per capita.

The number of ESRD patients per million population on therapy in Eastern Europe was 40% of that in Western Europe. Only patients with failure from primary renal causes (intrinsic renal disease) were selected, the average age for starting ESRD treatment was lower, mortality higher, and hepatitis B more frequent. Peritoneal dialysis and kidney transplantation were less often used than in Western Europe.

The limitations of RRT in Eastern Europe were caused by the low GNP per capita, weak economy and lack of sufficient foreign currency for the import of dialysis technology from the West.

II. Introduction

The Central and Eastern European countries, in the past called 'socialistic' (Bulgaria, Czechoslovakia, German Democratic Republic, Hungary, Poland and Yugoslavia) are far behind the USA, Japan and Western Europe (so called capitalistic states) in the number of patients treated by RRT, and its quality. The cause of this and the development of dialysis and transplant activity in these countries can be understood only if the following is also taken into account; 1) development of dialysis technology, 2) growth of dialysis and transplant activity in rich and developing countries, 3) economic strength of individual states, and 4) isolation of Eastern European countries during the 'cold' war.

189

C. M. Kjellstrand and J. B. Dossetor (eds): Ethical Problems in Dialysis and Transplantation, 189–200.
© *1992 Kluwer Academic Publishers. Printed in the Netherlands.*

III. Development of dialysis technology

Although the artificial kidney machine, employable for humans, was constructed as early as 1943 [1], it was the discovery of teflon, a biologically inert substance and its use for the construction of permanent arteriovenous shunts by Quinton and Scribner in 1960 that enabled repeated connection of patients to the artificial kidney [2]. Further progress came with the introduction of the subcutaneous arteriovenous fistula in 1966 [3].

The second major advance in regular dialysis treatment was replacement of bicarbonate by acetate in 1964 [4]. But the preparation of a dialysis machine was still very time-consuming [5]. The first factory-made dialysers, the coils, required large volumes of blood to prime them and had large residual blood volumes [5, 6]. They needed a blood pump to overcome resistance in the long cellophane tubes. The results of therapy were not as good as those obtained with Kiil's parallel-flow plate dialysers [7, 8, 9]. In 1968 Alwall [10, 11] devised the first factory-made parallel dialysers, and the firm Gambro entered the field to manufacture them (Table 1). By the beginning of the seventies, technological developments enabled regular dialysis treatment to be used widely.

Table 1. Development of dialysis technology

Year	Intervention	Author
1943	Rotating drum artificial kidney machine	Kolff [1]
1946	Alwall's artificial kidney	Alwall [10]
	Murray's artificial kidney	Murray [5]
1955	Twin coil artificial kidney	Watschinger, Kolff [6]
		Travenol
1960	Parallel flow artificial kidney	Kiil [7]
	Arterio-venous shunt	Quinton, Scribner [2]
1964	Substitution of sodium acetate for sodium	
	bicarbonate in the bath fluid	Mion [4]
1966	Subcutaneous arterio-venous fistula	Brescia, Cimino [3]
	Proportioning and monitoring systems	
1968	First factory made disposable	Alwall [11]
	parallel flow plate dialysers	Gambro [8]

IV. Growth of dialysis and transplant activity

A. *USA and Japan*

Hemodialysis treatment of ESRD patients was initiated in 1960 in Seattle by Scribner and co-workers [12]. Although data on dialysis activity in the whole of the USA have only been available since 1968 [13], regular dialysis treatment became

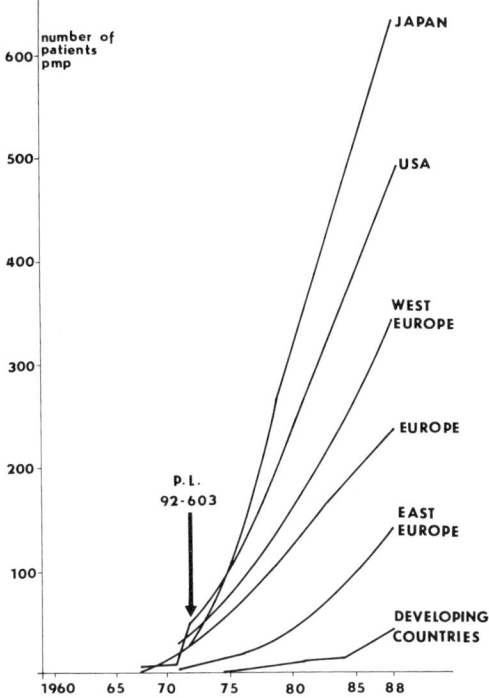

Figure 1. Growth of dialysis and transplant activity in USA, Japan, West Europe and developing countries around the Mediterranean Sea from 1960 to 1988.

most frequently used after 1973 when the U.S. Congress enacted law 92–603 which enabled dialysis costs, for all, to be fully met by the state. Home dialysis treatment, successfully developing until then, was not financially covered and started to stagnate. The proportion of patients treated by home dialysis decreased from 40% in 1972 to 12% in 1978. Since 1978, due to amendment of 95–292, full reimbursement of costs was approved for home dialysis treatment and an increase of home dialyses has been observed.

In 1988, 105,958 patients were on kidney dialysis in the United States. In the same year, 9123 kidney transplantations were performed [13].

Renal replacement therapy was developing similarly in Japan. For religious reasons, only a small fraction of patients were transplanted. Also peritoneal dialysis was seldom used.

If all patients treated by individual methods of RRT in USA are compared to patients on dialysis in Japan, approximately the same number of ESRD patients are on therapy in both countries, approaching 600 patients per million/population (see Figure 1).

192

B. *Europe and developing countries around the Mediterranean*

Regular dialysis treatment and kidney transplantation started in Europe in 1961, and ceased to be an experimental procedure. Since 1969 the pace of development has steadily increased. By 1988 an average of 232 patients per million were under treatment in Europe and the countries around the Mediterranean [6].

The rate at which the number of ESRD patients increased in different parts of Europe was very unequal. In 1988, 343 patients per million were treated on average in Western Europe, while there were only 142 in the Central and Eastern Europe, and 43 in developing countries around the Mediterranean (Algeria, Egypt, Lebanon, Libya, Morocco, Tunisia and Turkey) (see Figure 1).

Belgium was the leader among Western European countries with 447 patients per million and Greece trailed, with 203 (Figure 2). The ratio of difference between the first and last was 2.2:1. Among Eastern European countries, the difference was higher : 232 patients per million were treated in Yugoslavia and 70 in Poland (ratio 3.3:1) (Figure 3). In developing countries around the Mediterranean the ratio was as high as 5.5:1 (Tunisia: 94 patients; Morocco 17) [14].

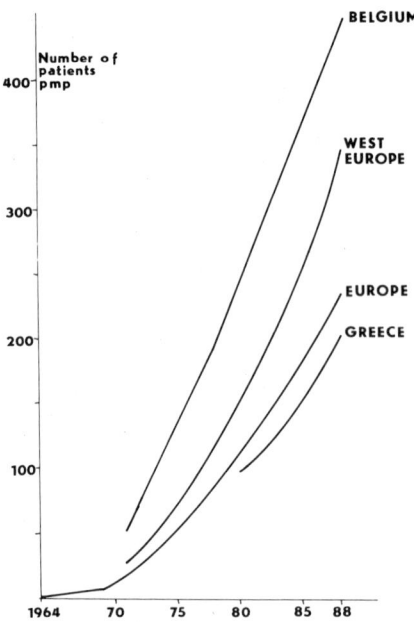

Figure 2. Development of renal replacement therapy in Europe and Western Europe on the average, and in the countries with the highest (Belgium) and lowest (Greece) number of patients.

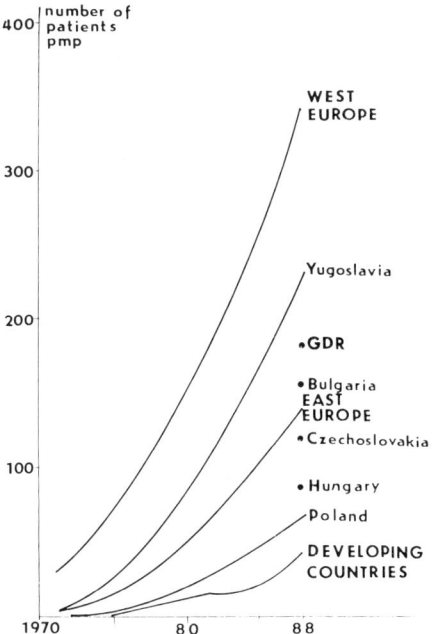

Figure 3. Development of renal replacement therapy in Eastern European countries.

V. The relationship between economic strength of the country and the number of patients on RRT (Figure 4)

Wing and co-workers showed in 1982 [15] that the GNP per capita relates to the number of patients on RRT. In countries with a GNP of less than $3,000 U.S. dollars per capita, dialysis and transplant activity is negligible. It is difficult and possibly even inappropriate for these countries to put many patients on treatment. In some countries with a low GNP per capita, priority is given to RRT in preference to other health care obligations and the number of patients is higher than the average. Eastern European countries belong to those in Europe with lower GNP per capita. In some of them, priority is also given to RRT (Yugoslavia, Bulgaria). Other countries are below the European average, but the number of patients is closely related to the GNP per capita [14–18].

VI. Quality of treatment

A. *Restriction in selection for RRT*

In a situation where dialysis technology is limited and not all patients with ESRD can be treated, a selection policy should be elaborated. The most reasonable policy

194

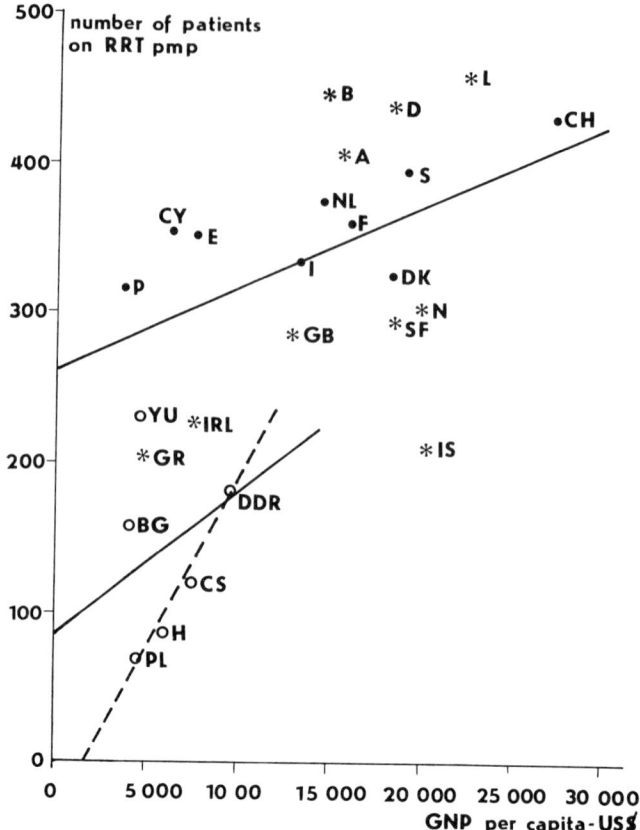

Figure 4. Relationship between the number of patients on renal replacement therapy per million and gross national product per capita in US dollars in 19 'West' and 'East' European countries.
'West Europe' : $r = 0.0581$, $y = 262 + 0.0054x$, $p > 0.05$;
'East Europe' : $r = 0.5976$, $y = 84.2 + 0.009x$, $p > 0.05$.
Countries marked with a star were one standard deviation above the line of correspondence and one standard deviation below. Iceland was two standard deviations below. Yugoslavia was one standard deviation above. Dashed line represents 'East' European countries, in which priority is not given to RRT and the number of patients corresponds to the gross national product per capita.
A = Austria, B = Belgium, BG = Bulgaria, CS = Czechoslovakia, CY = Cyprus, D = Federal Republic of Germany, DDR = German Democratic Republic, DK = Denmark, E = Spain, F = France, GB = Great Britain, GR = Greece, H = Hungary, CH = Switzerland, I = Italy, IRL = Ireland, IS = Iceland, L = Luxembourg, N = Norway, NL = Netherlands, P = Portugal, PL = Poland, S = Sweden, SF = Finland, YU = Yugoslavia.

is to accept patients with the best prognosis, or with the best chance of kidney transplantation outcome.

ESRD patients with primary renal diseases have a lower mortality rate and are more easily rehabilitated than patients with multi-system diseases. Survival rate of grafts and patients who received the first graft over the age of 55 years is lower than in younger age groups [16].

In Eastern Europe this was the basis for selection. In Western Europe, in 1987, new patients included 14.5% with diabetic nephropathy and 7.2% with multi-system disease, whereas in Eastern Europe, it was only 8.1% and 2.9%, respectively. In Northern and Western Europe, 27% grafts were transplanted at recipient age group of 55–64 years and 4% at 65–74 years, whereas in Eastern Europe it was only 4% and 0.2%, respectively. In Southern Europe, where transplantations of older age groups is not so frequent as in the North and West, these rates were still higher than in Eastern Europe (7% and 0.3%, respectively) [16]. The 'first come, first serve' lottery method was used.

B. *Death rates*

The cumulated first year mortality rate of hemodialysis fell from over 50% in patients started in 1965, to less than 15% in patients started in 1977 and 1978. This improvement occurred in spite of a sharp rise in the mean age for starting hemodialysis [19]. In Europe, the mortality rate of patients on RRT decreased from

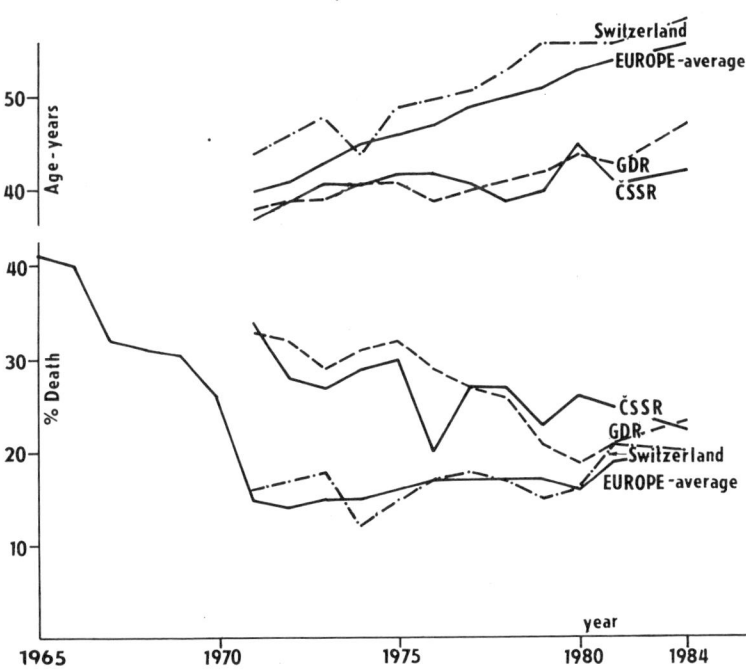

Figure 5: Mortality rate of patients and age at the start of dialysis therapy in Europe on an average, Switzerland, Czechoslovakia and German Democratic Republic.

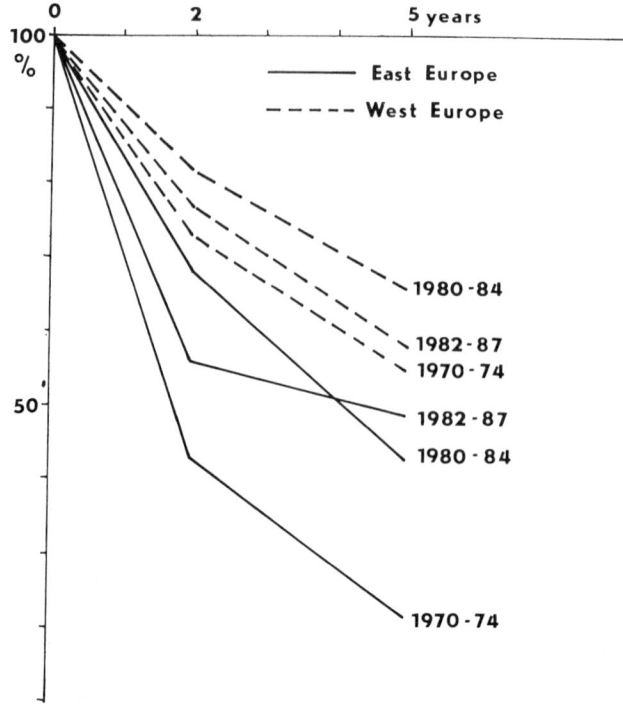

Figure 6. Per cent acturial survival of all patients starting renal replacement therapy 1970–1974, 1980–1984 and 1982–1987 in West/ dashed line/ and East Europe/ full line/.

41% in 1965 to 14% in 1972, but increased again to 19% in 1981. When mortality rates for 1972–1983 were compared with the age of starting dialysis, the mortality rate curve rises more steeply in relation to age, especially in the case of Switzerland, one of the foremost European countries to practice RRT, see Figure 5. It may be concluded that the increased mortality was caused by a higher proportion of older patients, but also the quality of dialysis improved so as partly to offset the associated rise in age-related mortality.

While the age for starting dialysis was 10–15 years lower in Czechoslovakia and the German Democratic Republic than in Switzerland, mortality rates were 10% higher. Mortality rate decreased substantially after 1975 in the German Democratic Republic, and after 1980 in Czechoslovakia. At this time, coil dialysers were changed for hollow fibre dialysers in GDR and for disposable plate dialysers in Czechoslovakia (Figure 5).

Per cent actuarial survival of patients starting RRT in 1970–74, 1980–84 and 1982–87 shows that survival rates in Eastern European countries were always lower than in Western Europe, even if they were approaching in the year 1980–84 and 1982–87 [14, 20] (Figure 6).

C. *Hepatitis B*

Incidence of hepatitis B was compared in Czechoslovakia and France as representative countries of Eastern and Western Europe. The number of new patients and staff with hepatitis B was twice as high in Czechoslovakia as in France. However, the incidence of hepatitis in staff rapidly decreased in 1987. Active immunization of patients and staff started in France in 1978, but in Czechoslovakia in 1986 only staff were immunized [21] (Figure 7).

D. *Home dialysis and transplantation*

Home dialysis and kidney transplantation are less expensive methods of RRT than hemodialysis.

Only 0.8% of all patients on dialysis were treated by home hemodialysis and 1.1% by peritoneal dialysis in Eastern Europe, while it was 4.3 and 17.3% respectively in the West. Four of six East European countries (Bulgaria, German Democratic Republic, Hungary and Poland) had no patients on home dialysis in 1988.

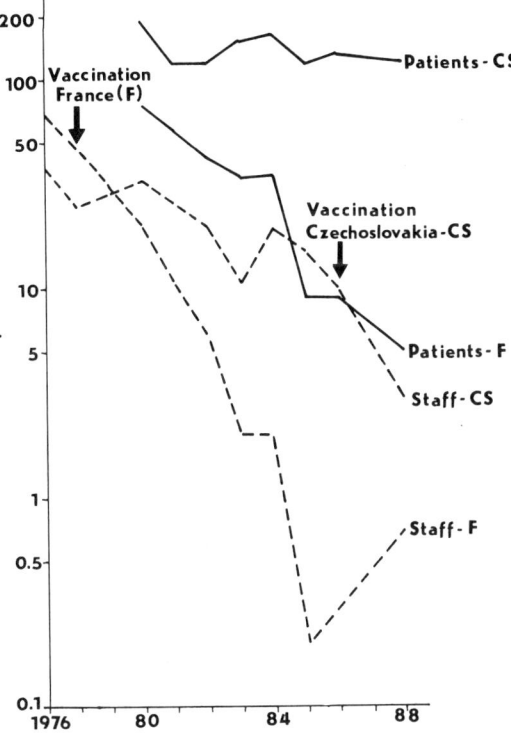

Figure 7. Incidence of hepatitis B in patients /P/ and staff /S/ in Czechoslovakia /CS/ and France /F/.

Resources for RRT in the United Kingdom are limited and that country's number of RRT patients per million is fourth from the bottom for Western Europe. The difference in less expensive methods of treatment was much greater than between 'East' and 'West' with 0.6% of patients on home dialysis in Czechoslovakia and 32% in United Kingdom, 1% and 47% respectively on peritoneal dialysis. This is remarkable as Czechoslovakia and Great Britain have comparable GNP per capita.

The proportion of ESRD patients alive with a functioning graft was 45% for Western Europe and 22% for Eastern Europe, with variation from 84% in Norway to 10% in Greece, and from 35% in Poland to 3% in Bulgaria in 1988.

A similar number of patients was on RRT in Czechoslovakia and Norway, but 1,365 were treated by hemodialysis in Czechoslovakia and only 174 in Norway. Up to six patients may be treated by one artificial kidney machine. Thus, Czechoslovakia would need 227 units, but Norway only 29 (Table II).

Table II. Proportion of patients alive with functioning graft or on hemodialysis in Norway and Czechoslovakia, in 1988.

1988	Total number of patients	With functioning graft	On hemodialysis	No. of artificial kidney machines
Norway	1226	1052	174	29
Czechoslovakia	1846	481	1365	227

High transplant activity in Norway and other Northern European countries is caused by their transplant policy. In Norway 39% of patients received grafts from living donors compared with only 1% in Czechoslovakia, in 1988. There were 55 patients per million in Czechoslovakia and 21 in Norway on the waiting list for cadaver kidney transplant [16].

VII. Causes of limited RRT in Eastern European countries

The development of RRT in USA has shown that there are two main preconditions for expansion of dialysis: technology and money. The increment of hemodialysis therapy started in the late sixties and early seventies when sophisticated technology became available and accelerated in 1973, when the US government started to cover all expenses.

In Eastern Europe the number of patients per million treated by RRT is lower than in the rich industrialized countries. Only patients with ESRD due to intrinsic renal disease are selected. Mortality rate is higher, incidence of hepatitis B more frequent, and home dialysis, peritoneal dialysis and kidney transplantation less often used than in the Western countries.

The GNP per capita in Eastern European countries is low and their economies are weak. They do not have enough of the so-called hard currency for import of dialysis technology: hemodialysis machines, dialysers, hemofilters, and peritoneal dialysis bags. On the other hand, all medical care which can be obtained by use of domestic currency is free and sufficient.

In the majority of dialysis centers in Eastern Europe six patients are treated with one artificial kidney machine, as each unit must be used as much as possible. Five patients on home hemodialysis in Czechoslovakia in 1988 were treated by older deteriorated machines which could no longer be used three times per day for seven days a week in the dialysis center, but could still function three times weekly in the home.

The hepatitis virus may pass across the membrane of dialysers from blood to dialysate. Using recirculated single pass hemodialysis machines and coil dialysers, aerosols contaminated by virus were found in the air of some dialysis centers. Moreover, it was very difficult to sterilize complicated dialysate systems. Hepatitis B active immunization is expensive and vaccines are not produced in Eastern European countries. They, too, must be imported from the West.

The lower number of patients living with functioning graft in Eastern Europe, especially in comparison with the Northern European countries, is explained by the lower number of patients, both on hemodialysis and on the waiting list for cadaver kidney transplant. An apparent exception to this, where Czechoslovakia had 55 patients per million on the waiting list in 1988, and Norway only 20, is due to the much higher proportion of living donors in Northern Europe and the higher transplantation rate in previous years due to their transplant policy.

Information about dialysis and transplant activity in the USSR and Rumania is not available. On the basis of personal experience, the number of patients on RRT per million is lower there than in any of the other Eastern European countries.

Eastern Europe is becoming less isolated and rejoining the rest of the developed world. Its economy will improve and it will obtain exchangeable currency. This may help in developing their programs for RRT, however, this anticipated economic growth will require great effort and will take time.

References

1. Kolff WJ. The artificial kidney. Past present and future. Circulation 1957; 15: 285.
2. Quinton W, Dillard D, Scribner BH. Cannulation of blood vessels for prolonged hemodialysis. Trans Amer Soc Artif Intern Org 1960; 6: 104.
3. Brescia MJ, Cimino JE, Appell K et al. Chronic hemodialysis using venipuncture and a surgically created arteriovenous fistula. New Engl J Med 1966; 275: 1089.
4. Mion CM, Hegstrom RM, Boen SI et al. Substitution of sodium acetate for sodium bicarbonate in the bath fluid for hemodialysis. Trans Am Soc Artif Intern Organs 1964; 10: 110.
5. Murray G, Delorme E, Thomas N. Development of an artificial kidney. Arch Surg 1947; 55: 505.
6. Watchinger B, Kolff JW. Further development of the artificial kidney of Inouye and Engelberg. Trans Am Soc Artif Intern Organs 1955; 1: 37.

7. Kiil F. Development of a parallel flow artificial kidney in plastics. Acta Chir Scand/Supp/ 1960; 253: 142.
8. Kjellstrand CM, Buselmeier TJ, Duncan D *et al*. A new disposable parallel flow artificial kidney/AB Gambro/. Comparison with the Ultraflo 100, 145 and the Kill. Proc Europ Dial Transpl Assn 1970; 7: 430.
9. Alberts Ch, Drukker W. Report on regular dialysis treatment in Europe: Proc Europ Dial Transpl Assn 1965; 2: 82.
10. Alwall N. A new disposable artificial kidney; experimental and clinical experiences: Proc Europ Dial Transpl Assn 1968; 5: 18 & 429.
11. Alwall N. On the artificial kidney I. Apparatus for dialysis of blood *in vivo*. Acta Med Scand 1947; 128: 317.
12. Scribner BH, Bari R, Caner JEZ *et al*. The treatment of chronic uremia by means of intermittent dialysis: a preliminary report. Trans Amer Soc Artif Intern Organs 1960; 6: 114.
13. Evans RW. Organ donation: facts and figures. Dialysis and Transplantation 1990; 19: 234.
14. Combined Report on Regular Dialysis and Transplantation in Europe, XIX, 1988, Nephrol Dial Transpl 1989; 4/ suppl 4/: 5.
15. Wing AJ, Selwood NH. Achievements and problems in the treatment of and stage renal failure. In Jones NF (ed) Recent advances in renal medicine. Peters DK 1982; 2: 103.
16. Brunner FP, Wing AJ, Dykes SR *et al*. International review of renal replacement therapy: strategies and results. In Maher JF (ed): Replacement of renal function by dialysis, 3rd edition. Dordrecht/Boston/Lancaster: Kluwer Academic Publishers, 1989; p. 697.
17. World Bank Atlas, Washington DC, World Bank, 1989.
18. Hinds M, McKinnon R, Simonian R. Perestroika. The Economist 1990; 315, 7652: 58.
19. Kjellstrand CM. Hemodialysis – The gold standard. Proc 9th Int Congr Nephrol, Athens 1981, University Studio, Thessaloniki, S Karger, Basel, 1981; p. 708.
20. Brunner FP, Broyer M. Brynger H *et al*. Survival on renal replacement therapy: Data from the EDTA registry. Nephrol Dial Transplant 1988; 2: 109.
21. Combined Report on Regular Dialysis and Transplantation in Europe XVIII, 1987. Nephrol Dial Transplant 1989; 4/ suppl. 2/: 5.

17. A different view from different countries: United Kingdom

A.J. WING

I. Introduction

The National Health Service (NHS) has, since 1948, provided medical services for all entitled people living in Great Britain (England, Scotland and Wales) and Northern Ireland. In the period of austerity following the second World War and at a time of relatively unsophisticated medical science the NHS was introduced to these island countries which together comprise the United Kingdom (U.K.). The aims of the sevice were that it should be free at the point of need and equally available to all socio-economic groups and in all parts of the U.K.

The people were beguiled by the State providing for their medical needs. The profession who staffed the service were at first privileged dispensers, operating in a realm of clinical freedom unfettered by financial constraint, and the politicians greedily accorded themselves the credit for the service known as the 'jewel in the crown of the Welfare State'. However, the people had been accustomed to rationing because they had recently been living in an island under siege. The professions had inherited a status in society which allowed them to adopt a paternalistic attitude to taking life and death decisions for an unquestioning public. The politicians believed their own rhetoric.

Into this society and onto the backs of such an idealistic health service was pitched all the ethical and economic challenge of high technology medicine, amongst which came dialysis and transplantation to offer life to patients dying of a rapidly fatal condition, end-stage renal failure (ESRF). This chapter relates how the NHS tried to meet this challenge, the indirect and subtle way in which rationing was enforced, the resulting pattern of therapy and triage-like selection of patients, and the ethical debate which has been provoked.

It is an interesting time to do such a review for the NHS is about the undergo a fundamental revolution in its ethos, and in 1991/2 is about to be turned to embrace the mechanisms of the marketplace, where bargain-hunting purchasers haggle with entrepreneurial providers. Will the new style NHS give the patient with ESRF a better deal? Will it change the strategy and scale of renal replacement therapy (RRT)?

201

C. M. Kjellstrand and J. B. Dossetor (eds): Ethical Problems in Dialysis and Transplantation, 201–226.
© 1992 *Kluwer Academic Publishers. Printed in the Netherlands.*

II. History of rationed treatment for ESRF under the NHS

A. *Pattern of RRT*

The pattern of treatment modalities which emerged under the peculiar restraints of the NHS is strikingly different from patterns in other countries [1]. The deployment of hospital hemodialysis, which is the mainstay of renal replacement therapy elsewhere, has been kept in check in the UK. Physicians have therefore had to turn to home hemodialysis in early years and continuous ambulatory peritoneal dialysis (CAPD) more recently, for maintenance therapy. As illustrated in Figure 1, from 1975 to '80 there were twice as many patients on home hemodialysis as were on hospital hemodialysis in the U.K. Commencing in 1979, CAPD made an increasingly significant contribution to independent dialysis and by 1985 there were more patients on this form of dialysis than on either home or hospital hemodialysis. As the contribution of CAPD grew, so home hemodialysis declined: by the close of 1987 more than twice as many patients carried out CAPD as performed hemodialysis at home. Rising above all dialysis modalities, renal transplantation became the single most important therapy in numerical terms from 1977 onwards [2]. No other European country (see Figure 2), and certainly none elsewhere in the world, has evolved a pattern of treatment modalities like that in the U.K. The uniqueness of the constraints and rationing mechanisms of the NHS must be held responsible [3].

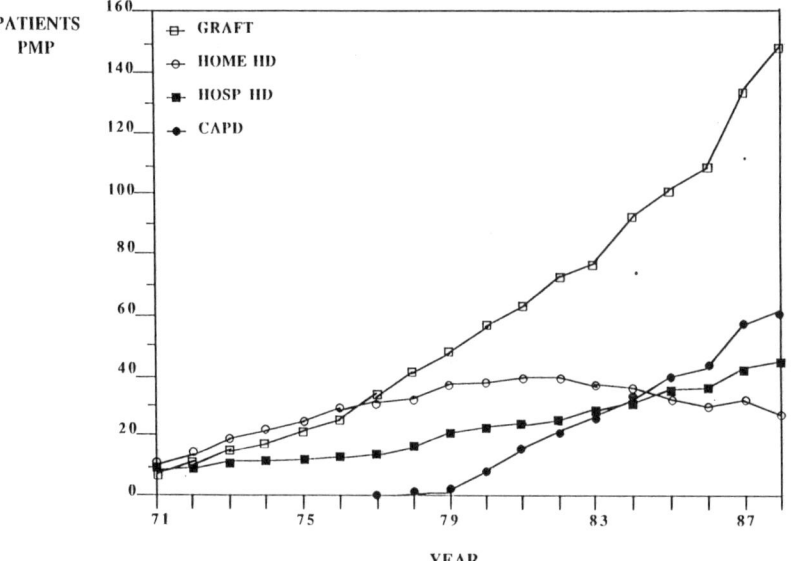

YEAR

Figure 1. Stocks of patients alive in U.K. on 31st of December in each of the years 1971 to 88 according to method of treatment. Numbers are given per million population (latest population of U.K. = 57.019 m). Figure from Wing [2], reproduced from advances in renal disease, Ed. AEG Raine by permission of Oxford University Press. Data from EDTA registry.

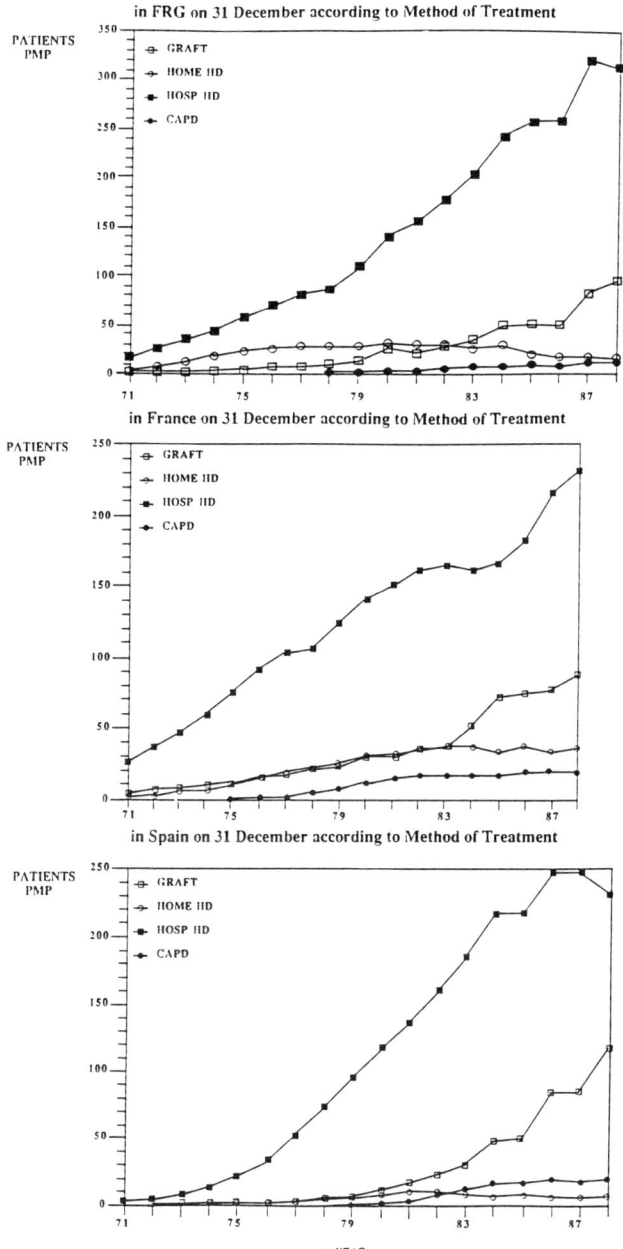

Figure 2. Stocks of patients alive (pmp) in the Federal Republic of Germany, France and Spain on 31st December in each of the years 1971–88 according to method of treatment. Numbers are given per million population (latest populations: FRG = 61.049, France = 55.873, Spain = 38.997). Note that the vertical scales are not identical. Data from EDTA Registry.

204

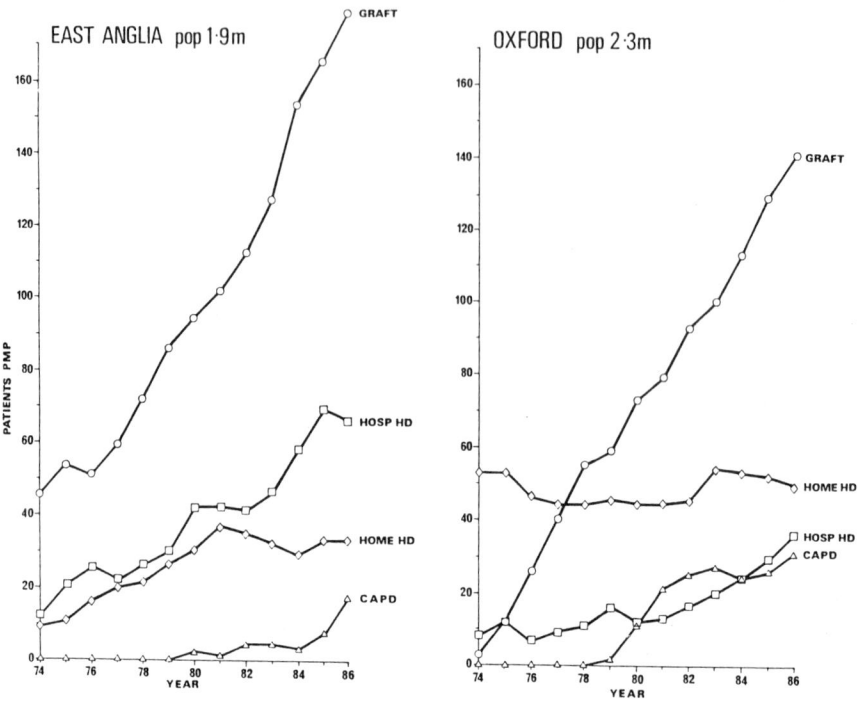

Figure 3. Stocks of patients alive (pmp) in two U.K. health regions. East Anglia and Oxford on 31st December in each of the years 1974–86. Data from EDTA registry.

However, the overall pattern for the UK conceals interesting regional variations [4]. Renal transplantation has been notably successful in the region of East Anglia in which the University of Cambridge, with a famous professorial unit for transplantation, is sited. Transplantation was introduced more recently in Oxford where previously home hemodialysis had been strongly developed (Figure 3). The large regions with a predominently metropolitan population in the South East of the country mirrored the U.K. pattern, but in the South West and in Yorkshire, the service for rural populations has relied heavily on home hemodialysis and CAPD. The regional patterns of treatment thus reveal the influence of the local population and the historic contributions of major units and personalities with the philosophies inherent in their different approaches.

These regional variations suggest that NHS constraints have not amounted to a straight-jacket since there has been sufficient flexibility in the system to allow individual variations. Nevertheless, the theme which emerges shows that the system encourages the development of transplantation and of independent methods of dialysis. Traditional British attitudes have probably eschewed forms of dialysis which make the patient permanently dependent on the hospital, and are therefore probably responsible in part for permitting the growth in numbers of hospital dialysis centres to have been so slow.

B. *Selection of patients*

Implicit in the U.K. strategy of RRT has been the attitude that patients who are incapable of performing independent dialysis or who are unlikely to be transplanted are less suitable for the treatment program available. This attitude has been sensed by physicians in the selection and referral chain with the result that high

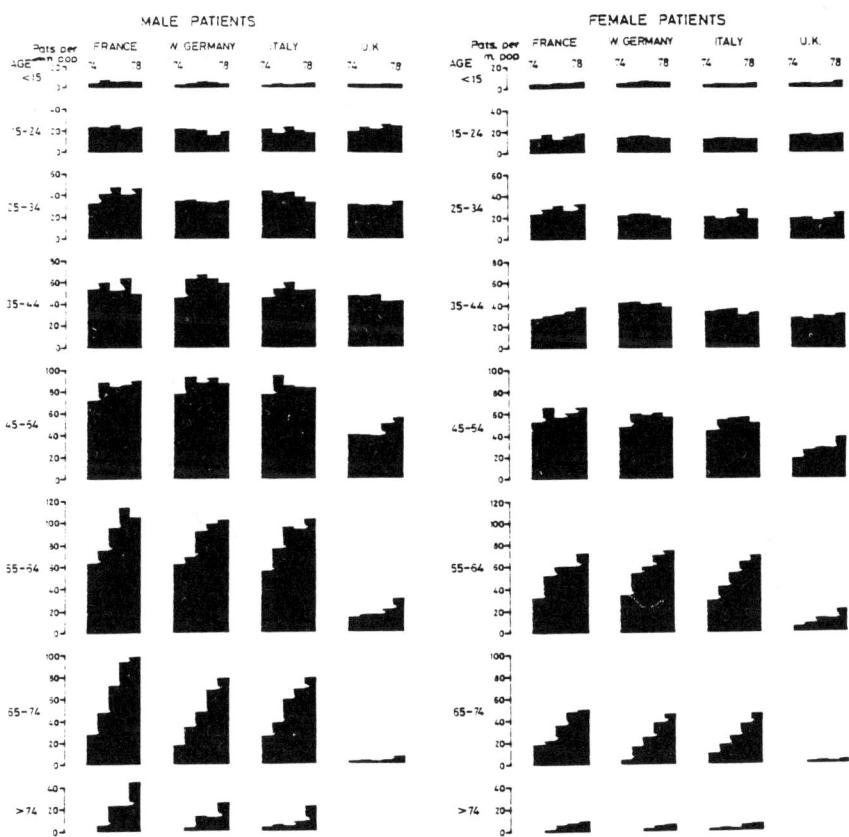

Figure 4. Age and sex specific new patient acceptance rate pmp in France, Federal Republic of Germany, Italy and U.K. 1974–78. Reproduced by permission of the editor of the proceedings EDTA.

risk patients, for example the elderly and the diabetic, have tended to be excluded [5].

It was the age and sex specific patient acceptance rates analyses performed by the EDTA Registry on 1974–78 data which drew attention to the striking difference between practices in three other large Western European countries (France, Federal Republic of Germany and Italy) and the U.K. (Figure 4). This early figure showed that the U.K. program was comparable with those in the other countries for patients aged up to 44, but that in the age range 45–54 for both male and female patients, the acceptance was lowest in the U.K. Patients aged over 55 had a poor chance of being taken onto treatment. This observation prompted an outspoken leading article

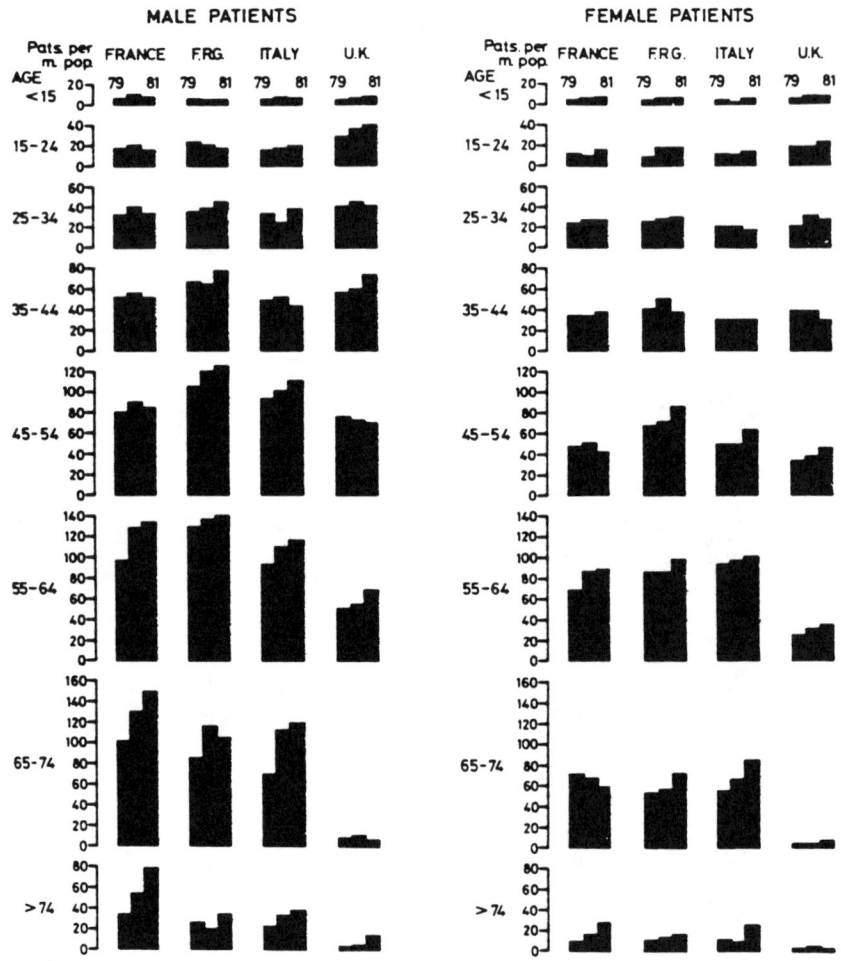

Figure 5. Age and sex specific new patient acceptance rate pmp in France, Federal Republic of Germany, Italy and U.K. 1979–81. Reproduced from the Oxford Text Book of epidemiology Ed W.W. Holland by permission of Oxford University Press.

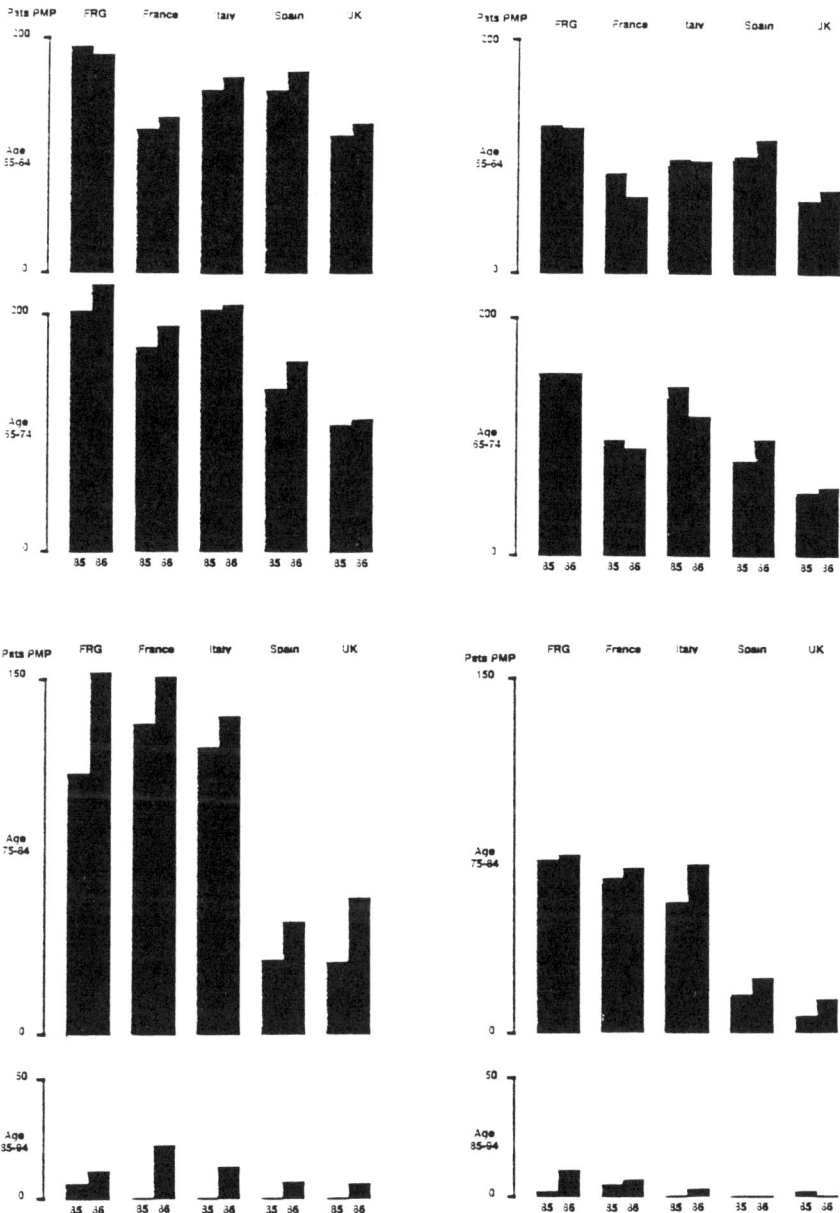

Figure 6. Age and sex specific new patient acceptance rate pmp in Federal Republic of Germany, France, Italy, Spain and U.K. for patients aged 55 to 94, 1985–86. Left panel = male patients; Right panel = female patients.

208

[6] which interpreted the data as the product of bureaucratic edict. Other authors have used the same figure to illustrate what they perceive as the iniquities of socialized medicine.

When the analysis was repeated on the subsequent three years data, 1979–81, the trend for increasing patient acceptance rates in the age ranges 45–54, 55–64 and over 65, which were only perceptible in the data for 1974–78, now showed that the catching up process was continuing although acceptance rates for patients aged 55–64 in the U.K. was still about half those in the other three countries [5].

The analysis has been repeated on 1985–86 data and results for patients aged over 55 are shown in Figure 6. On this occasion data for Spain were included. Acceptance rates in the U.K. for both male and female patients aged 55–64 were comparable with those in France but a little lower than those in Federal Republic of Germany, Italy and Spain. When patients in the age ranges 65–74 and 75–84 are considered it is at these ages that the U.K. now falls behind the other large Western European countries.

Taken together, these three analyses show how treatment programs in U.K. have progressively expanded to accommodate the older patients. In all years, the provision of treatment for children and young adults has been on a par with standards set elsewhere. This shows that the system for detecting ESRF and for arranging treatment can efficiently meet the needs of the younger population. It may be significant that the treatment of older patients was restrained until the 1980s because these were the years when CAPD became available [7].

Faced in the early 1980s with the fact that selection of patients was occurring, nephrologists claimed that they were not turning large numbers of patients away. Challah and colleagues [8] carried out a survey to investigate the question of under-referral. They sent a questionnaire comprising 16 case histories of patients with established ESRF and associated medical and social problems, to various groups of randomly chosen doctors throughout the country, and to selected nephrologists in other countries. In each case, the responding doctor was asked to

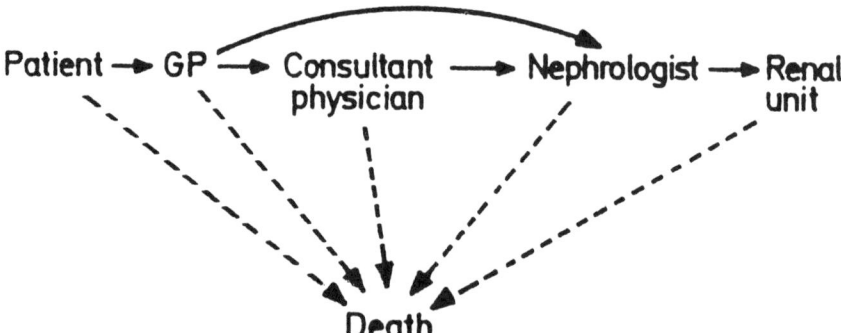

Figure 7. Referral pathway for patient developing chronic renal failure in United Kingdom. Reproduced from 8 by permission of the editor of the Brit Med J.

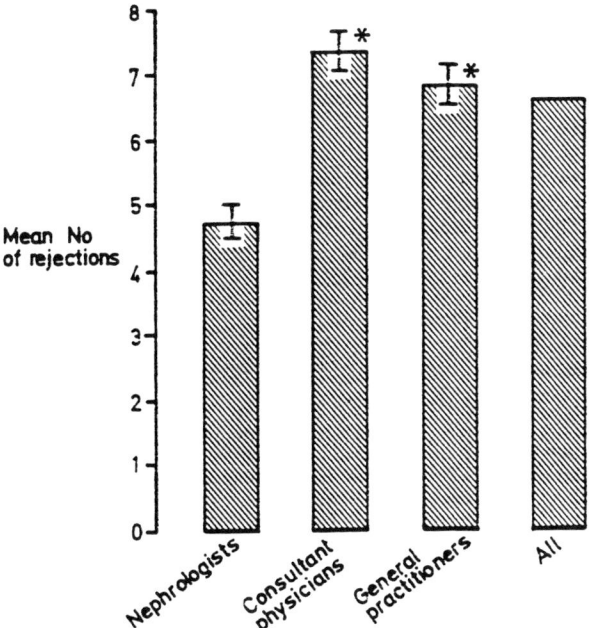

Figure 8. Mean numbers of cases rejected (out of 16) by types of doctors. Bars are SDs. * Compared with nephrologists, p = <0.001. Reproduced from 8 by permission of the editor of the Br Med J.

indicate whether the patient would be suitable for treatment by dialysis and transplantation.

The mean number of cases rejected by General Practitioners was 6.9 out of the 16 and by consultant physicians it was 7.4 (Figure 8). These rejection rates were surprisingly higher than those recorded by British nephrologists (4.7) and strikingly different to those for North America (0.3) and Western Europe (3.6), although not dissimilar to the 7.5 of Eastern European returns. Rejection rates for individual cases varied from 8.4% for a 55 year old Jamaican woman with asthma to 83.9% for a 52 year old alcoholic man living in a hostel, who had failed to comply with therapy for hypertension. A striking observation was that among all groups of doctors the two cases with the lowest rejection rates were the same -namely, the 55 year old asthmatic and a 72 year old vet (Table I), suggesting that selection was based on general societal values rather than specialist insights.

The authors quote extensively from correspondence received with the returns because this was particularly revealing. It showed that decisions about whether or not patients with ESRF received treatment are often made in the U.K. without referral to a specialist, whereas this would be unusual in other countries. A decision to 'negatively select' would often be influenced by well publicised scarcity of facil-ities, and sometimes by a personal experience which was obviously out of date. It

Table 1. Percentages of various types of doctor rejecting each of 16 patients in questionnaire. Number in parentheses are ranking of cases (from 1 to 16) for rejection

Case No	Description of patient	Nephrologists	Consultant physicians	General practitioners
1	55 year old woman with asthma	1.1 (1)	9.2 (1)	10.7 (1)
2	72 year old male vet	4.4 (2)	18.4 (2)	19.1 (2)
3	36 year old man with paraplegia	7.7 (3)	18.9 (3)	26.5 (5)
4	53 year old male diabetic	9.9 (4)	23.2 (4)	37.7 (8)
5	59 year old female diabetic	16.5 (5 =)	41.1 (9)	41.9 (9)
6	25 year old blind male diabetic	16.5 (5 =)	28.7 (5)	23.3 (4)
7	62 year old man with stroke	20.9 (7)	50.3 (10)	45.1 (10)
8	49 year old woman with rheumatoid arthritis	22.0 (8)	31.9 (7)	28.4 (6)
9	50 year old educationally subnormal woman	23.1 (9)	40.5 (8)	36.3 (7)
10	45 year old female analgestic abuser	25.3 (10)	56.8 (11)	54.4 (11)
11	67 year old Asian with no English	26.4 (11)	30.8 (6)	22.3 (3)
12	51 year old woman with breast cancer	27.4 (12)	56.8 (12)	65.1 (13)
13	50 year old man with ischaemic heart disease	45.1 (13)	89.7 (15)	73.5 (15)
14	30 year old man with schizophrenia	58.2 (14)	71.9 (13)	56.7 (12)
15	52 year old male alcoholic	79.1 (15)	90.3 (16)	80.5 (16)
16	29 year old hepatitis B positive man	86.8 (16)	85.4 (14)	71.6 (14)

seems particularly likely that patients would be denied a nephrologist's opinion when this was not available locally.

C. *Referral practices*

Patients have no right to arrange their own appointments to see a consultant nephrologist. They must be referred by their General Practitioners who are now therefore regarded as the gatekeepers to the hospitals. They have limited access to investigatory facilities and so the diagnosis of advanced renal failure is probably made after referral to a hospital consultant. Rules governing referral and waiting times for consultation may delay diagnosis of renal failure. Firstly, there is a wide spectrum of symptoms, indeed, serious but gradually advancing renal failure is not infrequently without symptoms. This is notably the case in older patients for whom alternative explanations for non-specific symptomatology readily suggest them-selves. Secondly, progression over the final stages of uremia is often quite rapid. According to recent surveys, over half of the patients who had reached plasma creatinine concentration of 500 umols/l or urea concentrations of 25 mmols/l were either undergoing RRT or were dead within three months [9, 10]. Most British renal units report that about a third of patients who arrive in ESRF do so as acute uremic emergencies.

Entry to hospital through the emergency department is an alternative to a GP referral, but four out of every five District General Hospitals (which provide emergency services) do not have a renal unit or a nephrologist on their staff. Routine biochemistry in these hospitals does not always include the determination of creatinine. Referral to a renal centre is therefore often delayed, and I know of occasions when the delay proved fatal. Any doubt as to the suitability of the patient for RRT would add to delay during the referral process.

Why don't patients and their families ask for a second opinion? The answer to this is complex, and is not to be found in medical literature [11]. Although a patient has a very clear right to a second opinion, this is seldom requested. In Britain, a patient's attitude to his family doctor is generally trusting and deferential – 'he knows what is best'. Doctors are likely to adopt protective, even paternalistic attitudes. For most patients, referral to a hospital consultant is such a rare experience that it signals dire gloom, and it is naturally a great relief to be told that it is not necessary. For painful, obviously disabling diseases the system is satisfactory: pressing symptoms ensure appropriate action. However, uremia is uncommon, painless, insidious and, particularly in the elderly, accompanied by symptoms in other systems, notably cardiovascular, which can be treated. It is perhaps not too surprising that the patient and his family do not challenge what the primary physician believes.

D. *Numbers of centres and of nephrologists*

The crucial element in rationing dialysis in Britain has been the small number of centres [3]. Britain has 1.3 renal units per million population; in large Western European countries units tend to be smaller but they are more plentiful and evenly spaced. France reports 4.4 per million, Spain 5.6, Federal Republic of Germany 6.3, and Italy 7.1 [12]. Whereas the numbers of units has grown throughout the last two decades in these other countries, in the U.K. it has virtually stood still (Figure 9). How were the pressures to increase facilities resisted by the NHS?

The answer lies in the stranglehold of the bureaucratic machine but this is effectively camouflaged by the mechanisms through which it operates. Initially in the 1960s the NHS responded imaginatively to the challenge to set up dialysis facilities. This was the decade of burgeoning economies, of putting a man on the moon, and of high expectations of medical advances. In 1966, the Department of Health and Social Security (DHSS) set aside money centrally to establish one major centre in each region (population 1.8 to 5.2 million). Central funding like this is a most unusual practice but was done 'to get treatment established as quickly as possible and on a national basis' [13]. These units were regarded as 'nuclei for the further expansion of the service'. The short honeymoon came to an end in 1967 when financial responsibility was passed to regional boards because it was felt to be right that local authorities should 'have control over development and should decide themselves on priorities'. This can now be seen as an inevitable rationalization of

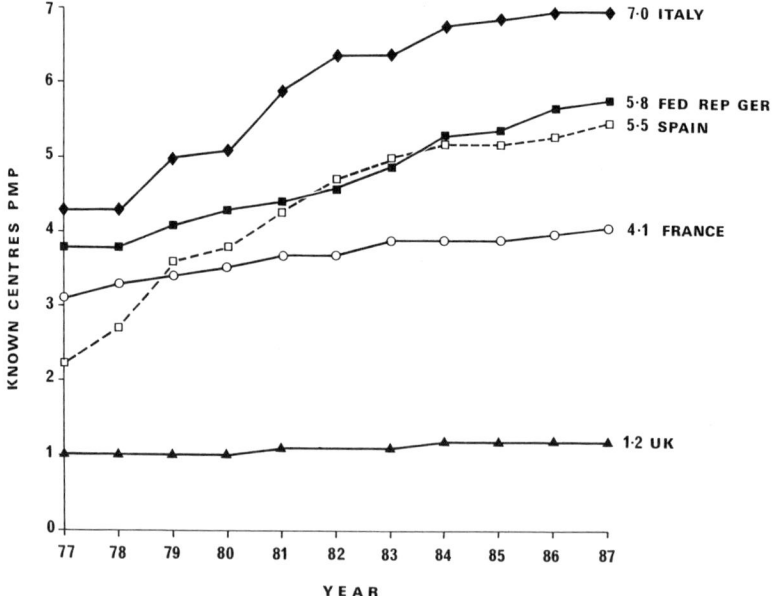

Figure 9. The number of renal units per million of population in 5 large Western European countries, 1977–87.

central authority's position since it could not accept the revenue implications of the capital expenditure which it had made. At that time capital investment in new services which was not backed by enhanced revenue to provide the running costs was beginning to be regarded as an unwelcome gift. On a smaller scale, nephrologists to whom dialysis machines were donated by charities would be discouraged from accepting them unless the full running costs, consumables, staffing and overheads were also donated. Regional authorities had just discovered the full cost implications of setting up new renal units and became resistant to proposals for further developments.

Hand in hand with the small number of units goes the small number of nephrologists. Other hospital consultants became aware of the resource commitment required to establish new posts for nephrologists, and when opportunities arose to make appointments, did not canvass strongly for this new specialty to be represented on their staff. Without a consultant nephrologist to collect his patients and make his case new renal units were very unlikely to become established. For readers to whom the workings of the NHS are strange it must be pointed out that a specialist, however well qualified and acknowledged even nationally or internationally, is effectively debarred from practicing as a specialist in the NHS until he or she has been appointed to an established consultant post with control over beds and other resources.

The result: Britain has only 1.5 whole time equivalent (WTE), senior staff (NHS consultants and academic staff with consultant status) practising nephrology per million of population. This does not bear comparison with other countries where five to ten times this number have access to treatment of their patients in a dialysis unit. Four surveys of manpower in adult renal medicine in the U.K. have been carried out by Jones and his colleagues, [14] on behalf of the Renal Disease Committee of the Royal College of Physicians and the Renal Association. They found that in 1975 there were 57 WTE senior staff each treating around 60 patients with ESRF; by 1989 this had grown by 30 WTEs and the 87 were each responsible for an average of nearly 200 patients (Figure 10).

The porportion of the population with insurance or personal means adequate to cover dialysis is negligible. Several small independent dialysis facilities have been opened, mostly in London, but they have failed to contribute significantly to NHS patients and are used almost exclusively for visitors not entitled to use the NHS, and particularly in preparation for transplantation. These facilities and the entrepreneur doctors who work in them could be commissioned to work for NHS patients, but until now funds have not been released for this purpose.

A study in the North West Thames region showed that rates of acceptance of new patients and of treatment were inversely related to the distance between patients' homes and the renal unit [15]. Patients with renal failure whose nearest renal unit is a long way from their home are disadvantaged and less likely to be treated. This observation is supported by data from North Devon and Blackburn where referral rates from centres of population without a renal unit were significantly lower than those from Exeter (South Devon), where there is a unit. Likewise in an urban population in London, South East Thames Regional Health Authority found highest take-on rates (124 pmp in Camberwell and 88 pmp in West Lambeth) in those districts in which renal units are situated. The message is

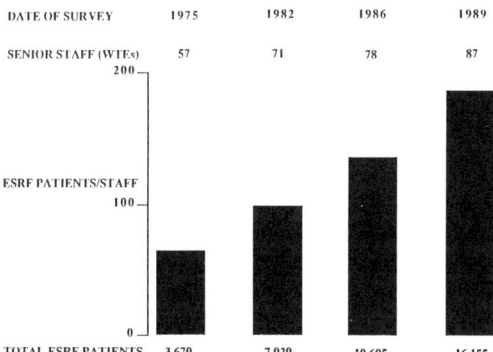

Figure 10. Manpower and workload in adult renal medicine in U.K. 1975–89. The relationship between numbers of senior staff in whole time equivalents and total ESRF patients alive on RRT is given for surveys carried out in 1975, 82, 86 and 89. Data from Jones *et al.* [14]. Reproduced from advances in renal medicine, Ed AEG Raine with permission of Oxford University Press.

214

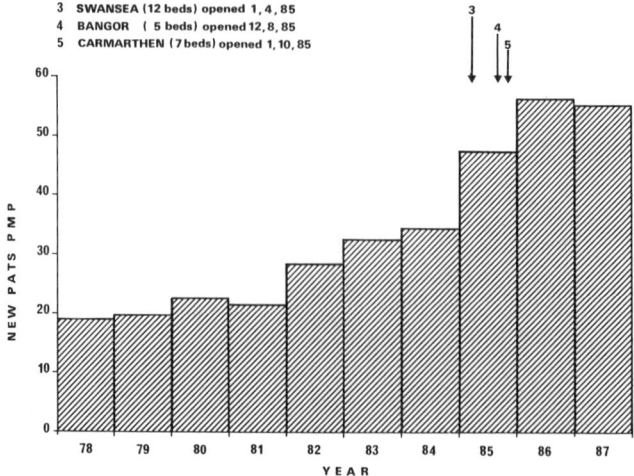

Figure 11. Annual acceptance rate for new patients pmp in Wales 1978–87. Note the effect of opening one new main renal unit in Swansea and two new subsidiary renal units in Bangor and Carmarthen in 1985.

obvious, new renal units should be placed in those areas with the lowest treatment rates.

This has been done in Wales. Two 'subsidiary' and one 'main' renal unit were added in 1985 to the two centres serving a population of 2.8 million [16]. Before these new units were opened the annual take-on rate in Wales was 34 pmp, after their commissioning the rate rose rapidly to over 60 pmp by 1987 (Figure 11).

Other arguments support the drive to open more centres and to appoint more nephrologists in order to fill the gaps in geographical provision. Patients are beginning to vocalize their wish to be treated nearer to home, preferably in smaller, more personal units. The high cost of transportation to remote units is borne by other budgets, but when this is noticed it will add powerful support on economic grounds.

E. *Negotiations to improve the service*

Over the decade of the eighties, representatives of the profession and successive Ministers of Health have engaged in a constructive dialogue about the level of services for dialysis and transplantation. The two sides were brought together through the officers of the All Party Disablement Group of the House of Commons. This group consists of Members of Parliament of all political persuasions. Discussions were founded on early studies of the number of patients needing treatment for ESRF. These studies were carried out in Northern Ireland [17], Scotland [18] and Wales [19] in the late 60s, and all yielded similar results, suggesting that taking an upper age limit of 60, there were about 40 new patients per million population who reached ESRF each year who should be treated. By 1982 the U.K. accepted 19.1 new patients pmp compared with 44 in West Germany and 41.3 in Sweden (Table II).

Table II. Acceptance of new patients pmp in European countries in 1982 and 1988. Data from EDTA registry

	Acceptance of new dialysis patients in Europe Quoted as numbers per million population per year	
Year	*1982*	*1988*
Austria	38.1	95.7
Belgium	39.6	85.2
Israel	58.2	80.0
West Germany	44.0	77.0
Holland	27.4	65.3
Sweden	41.3	64.3
Switzerland	44.5	61.8
Greece	18.8	59.2
Spain	32.7	57.1
France	30.9	56.3
Britain	19.9	55.1
Italy	33.8	54.7
Norway	37.3	52.7
Denmark	26.9	52.5
Ireland	19.4	33.8

This distressing comparison between the rates of treatment in U.K. and in other European countries [8] resulted in the Minister announcing on 20th December, 1984 an official policy of a target of 40 new patients pmp which all regions would be expected to achieve 'by 1987' [20]. On being questioned he replied that the target should be reached by 1st of January 1987, that is during the 12 months of 1986 in the regions which had already made most progress, whereas those who were significantly behind would be expected to achieve the target during the 12 months of 1987. This was a highly significant precedent, instituting for the first time a mechanism whereby a political decision of central government to provide a particular quota of therapy could be transmitted as a priority for regional health authorities. Thus national policy overruled local priority settings. It was implemented by regions 'top slicing' funds for ESRF treatment which were passed down to health districts on condition of fulfillment of their targets.

This in turn provoked heated discussions between regional authorities and health districts in which renal units were sited as to the true costs to be identified and reimbursed. The NHS did not have the mechanisms to cost individual patient therapys, and regions made mistakes in defining which costs should be included in adding up the total costs for RRT. For instance, should the costs of angioplasty and of hip replacement or of a pregnancy in a patient on RRT be included? The districts argued that they should because all the costs of treatments would be borne by the district providing the dialysis and transplantation which had kept alive a patient who would otherwise have died rapidly of uremia. Imprecise definitions lay behind the wide differences in costs reported for the five districts in the South East Thames region (Table III). Incredibly, these different costs were used for reimbursement pending agreement on 'standard costs'. Inevitably, this was frustrated by 4 out of the 5 units which would have had a reduction in reimbursement [4]. In the meantime, reimbursements varied by as much as 100%.

Table III. Cost of each of the modes of RRT in 5 centres serving the population of South East Thames Regional Health Authority

SETRHA experience: UNIT COSTS 87/88 Mode of Therapy	Regional Average (Range) – £s
Home haemodialysis	8,766 (6,664 – 25,583)
Hospital haemodialysis	15,930 (11,068 – 22,363)
CAPD	9,522 (6,037 – 14,050)
Transplant ops	5,610 (2,267 – 6,516)
1st Year's maintenance	5,545 (1,603 – 7,602)
Subs. year's maintenance	1,347 (250 – 2,125)

The Renal Association's response to the Minister's target was to carry out a study to predict the resources needed to implement this policy [21]. Using patient survival data from the EDTA registry, and information on in-patient facilities and staffing from the North Western Region, a scale of services which would be required for a steady state mathematical model was developed. One of the least noted but more alarming facts to come out of the study was the observation that a program for a region of 4 million inhabitants would require 45 in-patient beds – almost half the acute medical facilities of a small district general hospital.

The profession continued to be concerned by the poor performance of the U.K. and sponsored further studies of the rate of preventable deaths due to renal failure in Northern Ireland [9] and in Devon and Blackburn [10]. These studies, published in 1990 suggested that the real target should be 75 to 80 new patients pmp per year. It was the next stage in the dialogue for the Minister to accept the validity of these figures, which he did in 1990.

However, in the meantime a revolution in the administration and resourcing of the NHS was being planned.

F. *The 'new NHS'*

Monetarist policies, sometimes known as Thatcherism, are causing fundamental changes in the ethos of service provision in the U.K. How will this affect renal services? Instead of receiving a negotiated budget modulated in recent years by achievement targets, renal units will now become 'providers' selling their services to 'purchasers'. The purchasers are not the individual patients backed by insurance reimbursement but are the health districts who are responsible for buying services on behalf of the population of their areas. The amount of money which the districts have is determined by a capitation calculation which takes some account of demographic factors such as age distribution and level of social deprivation of their populations. Adjustment to this method of distribution of resources will be gradual, taking into account historic levels of health service usage.

The obvious danger is that purchasers will be attracted to the cheapest providers. It is hoped that patient choice will correct this tendency by influencing purchaser decisions. Choice will be influenced by the quality of care and attempts will be made to define this in contract agreements. Audit, outcome assessment and the discipline of contracts are intended to correct any trend towards the provision of inferior services. Difficulty in measuring the quality of clinical care is universally admitted. As we stand on the threshold of this new system the purchasers have not advanced beyond discussing waiting times for clinical appointments and for hospital admission. It is quite possible that one day they will want to define optimum biochemical control and hemoglobin levels but the complexities of case mix and difficulties in defining acceptable standards of care are likely to make such refinements unachievable in the foreseeable future.

The Government White Paper (a white paper is for implementation, not discussion) which introduced the new NHS was called 'Working for Patients' and was redolent with the expression 'Money will follow Patients' [22]. Renal physicians reacted favourably to the implication that an increase in work rate would attract more funding. It has also seemed likely to us that health districts might review existing patient flows and instead of commissioning remote renal units to treat their patients, might consider opening new facilities nearer to deprived centres of population. In this way market forces would naturally result in an increase in renal units and in numbers of nephrologists, reversing the uniquely constrained pattern of care described above [3]. We were encouraged in this thinking by the political statement that money which follows patients would make bureaucratic logjams simpler to resolve [23]. Our cautious enthusiasm for the new NHS is likely to be tempered by the overall limitation of money available. We are told that there will be no new money, and are alarmed that anticipated costs of new administration and of information technology will erode resources available for treating patients.

III. The ethical impact of rationed treatment for ESRF under the NHS

A. *The growing dilemma of financing healthcare*

Resources available for healthcare are not unlimited. Currently, the U.K. has available less than US $500 per year per person – under 7% of its per capita gross domestic product (GDP). In comparison, the USA spends two and a half times as much on healthcare around US $1300 per year, per person. Wages are lower in the

U.K. but the cost of equipment and consumables used for dialysis are similar. This would tend to make hemodialysis in U.K. relatively expensive, transplantation perhaps less so.

There is political pressure from medical professionals and patient support groups alike to increase the proportion of GDT spent on health. Increase in health expenditure is driven by five main factors – the altered pattern of diseases in increasingly elderly populations, advances in medical technology, increased expectations, rising manpower costs and progressive Government involvement to eliminate unacceptable inequalities [24]. It was observed over ten years ago that as health budgets reach above 10% of GDP the inevitable clash with other political priorities forces governments to apply the brakes on health expenditure [25]. It is now accepted as inevitable that countries will exercise some control over health care expenditure; but the question is how?

Various mechanisms exist to limit expenditure on medical services. Fiscal policy impacts on available individual wealth, employment arrangements affect insurance funding. Facilities can be restricted by licensing policies, planning procedures and budgetary control. Ultimately the reality of the high cost of RRT comes home to roost. To coin a phrase, there is no such thing as a free dialysis. Dialysis and transplantation have all the attributes of a medical intervention set to be a nightmare for health economists [5]. They make the difference between life and death – often for relatively young sufferers; they have reliable outcomes – with percentage survivals and quality of life matched by few treatments of rapidly fatal diseases; they are very expensive – and it is not just a one off expenditure, but costs are ongoing, the programs' annual bill expanding with the addition of every life it saves and continues to support.

Nephrologists cannot remain indifferent to the ethical problem they have posed for the societies which they serve. Those who specialized in nephrology in its early years were generally brave, pioneering physicians who did all they could to treat as many patients as possible with the limited facilities at their disposal. Inevitably they had to put pressure on their patients, operating a style of therapy which was epitomized by the expression 'go home or die'. Doctors felt guilt at doing this. They bore other burdens '... the physician gazing down at a young diabetic with progressive renal disease while he holds in his pocket a memo from the finance officer telling him that his budget is overspent, and while the pleas of the nursing sister in charge of his unit for "no more patients, please, because our nurses are on their knees, at breaking point and they will crack if I ask more of them" ring in his ears...' [26].

Guilt and the burden have taken their toll, and early death and morbidity is already detectable amongst my colleagues.

The conflict resulting from finding oneself the instrument of rationing when one had started out excited at new vistas of life saving potential, causes many of us to become active advocates of the patients, rejecting moral claims of our monopolistic employer, the State. Cameron and his colleages [27], in commenting on a much publicized attempt by the West Midlands region to cash limit its nephrologists, argued: 'as the patient's only advocate, the doctor is bound to do everything in his power to ensure that the patient in front of him gets the treatment he needs'. Later, Cameron threatened to use entry on death certificates to draw attention to inadequate treatment facilities. However, doctors do not easily resort to using the lives and deaths of individual named patients as political pawns. Media often request names in order to make an emotionally charged news item, shocking to viewers and readers, and designed to disturb the complacency of politicians and administrators [11]. Some of us began to feel that these 'shroud-waving' activities were sometimes demeaning of the profession, and risked overplaying the life and death context of RRT. We were not unaware of the needs of other groups of patients and of the wider context of the ethical impact of financial constraint [28]. Societies confront tragic choices when the affirmation of fundamental societal values is jeopardized by the conflict with scarcity of resources [29]. The challenge of making RRT available on a large scale presented this choice for the first time in the starkest terms. On the one hand, adoption of a polarized stance as the patient's advocate is the appropriate answer in a society in which decisions are thrashed out in adversarial debate. This risks the outcome that society may conclude that it must take the hard decisions on behalf of the professionals '...doctors will always spend everything we give them'. On the other hand, if we show ourselves balanced and objective, society may decide that the best person to make the difficult decision is the doctor, entrust to him a limited quantum of the nation's wealth and look to him to decide and to act ethically in the context of his acute conflict of interests.

Decisions about the allocation of resources have to be taken at two levels, the micro – and macro – allocative [30]. Doctors are obviously appropriate decision makers at the micro allocative level in which choice between patients and between interventions depends on clinical skills. They may also become increasingly involved in macro allocative decisions at a hospital, district, region and national level. As the scale of size is ascended, so physicians' ethical abilities are more critically tested. Decisions between competing claims must somehow take more information, data and propaganda into consideration, and come up with the right decision.

Under the new NHS, doctors are becoming more intimately involved in the management of budgets. This is an essential ingredient of the White Paper and independent or 'trust' status is being conferred on only those hospitals which can demonstrate that consultants play a real role in management. Clinicians are taking on the role of doctor-managers, budget holders, clinical directors and members of hospital executives and boards. As such they cannot align themselves with one group of patients alone but must face up to considering all sides in any conflict and then be accountable for their decision in the matter. Many nephrologists have been entrusted these roles by their colleagues and this bears testimony to the particular challenge and training of their specialty. It is a microcosm of the reality of making decisions in a resource limited environment.

B. *Decision taking in the renal unit*

Limited resources have forced us to practice triage. Patients who may become highly dependent requiring their treatment to be carried out by others, using more in-patient bed days and obligating elaborate community support, are likely to be 'negatively selected' [8]. High dependency is often equated with low quality of life. Harsh decisions are frequently rationalized on the grounds that to force a patient into a dependent role is to add to his suffering. At the worst, little thought is being given to the fact that we are brutalized by this process of cheapening life. We are at risk of becoming so appalled by the impossibility of funding a growing workforce to support these patients that we allow the status quo to pass as acceptable. But at the best we will rise to the challenge and develop the most cost effective forms of treatment and try very hard to restore independence to unlikely patients. Exciting examples of this are the widespread success of CAPD in U.K. and the expanding range of patients given transplants.

Limited resources are opening our eyes to non-economic practices. When dialysis has been costed in U.K. it has usually turned out to be more expensive than in USA. There is no doubt that hospital hemodialysis facilities are under used [31]. Reuse of dialysers, considered a sensible economy in USA has been declining in the U.K. [32]. Across the country we make too little use of dialysis assistants, employing probably too many skilled relatively highly paid nurses. It is hoped that the element of competition to be introduced by the new NHS will not only disclose non-economic practices but motivate practitioners to change them.

Limited resources are forcing hospital specialists into alliance with general practitioners. Budgetary constraints have induced us to consider all possible alternatives to funding. A doctor who manages the budget for a renal unit will soon become impressed by the large element of non-pay items for which he is paying. Financing the purchase of dialysis consumables, immunosuppressive drugs and erythropoietin competes with paying the wages of doctors, nurses, dieticians and other assistants. Unusual for hospital practice, non pay items exceed pay. The thought of firing medical staff in order to finance expenditure on erythropoietin presents a difficult decision and some units have had to withdraw the drug [33]. One solution has been to request general practitioners to prescribe the drugs and supplies so that they are transferred to their prescribing budget. Sensibly, the general practitioner is reluctant to do this unless he retains some clinical responsibility for the care of the patient. This has prompted an improved flow of information concerning the patient and his treatment from the hospital to the general practitioner, a development which can only be to the patient's advantage because it brings better informed assistance nearer to hand. It is also to the advantage of the general practitioner, who is no longer excluded from the 'high-tech' scene, and can now enter into important decisions such as whether or not his patients should opt for transplantation. These decisions may be influenced by the domestic environment which he knows best.

This movement of clinical responsibility back towards the general practitioner is consistent with the ethos of the new NHS. It is intended that ultimately, general practitioners will influence the use of resources by becoming budget holders and that through their budgets will exercise choice between hospital specialists and facilities. The gatekeepers will have the key placed in their hands.

C. Dialysis and transplantation versus other priorities

Figure 12 is the latest published [34] version of the correlation we have made between the numbers of patients treated by dialysis and transplantation and the wealth of individual countries. The correlation is highly significant and emphasises that the patient's chance of treatment depends on the wealth of the society to which he belongs. The correlation sustains its significance despite differences in the philosophy and delivery of health care in all these countries. Economic reality overrules political idealism. Saddest of all, those countries whose wealth creation is below US \$3000 per capita per year treat a negligible numbers of patients. This is not because their population suffer less from ESRD; they probably have more of it. Three-quarters of the world's population live in these poorer countries and for them

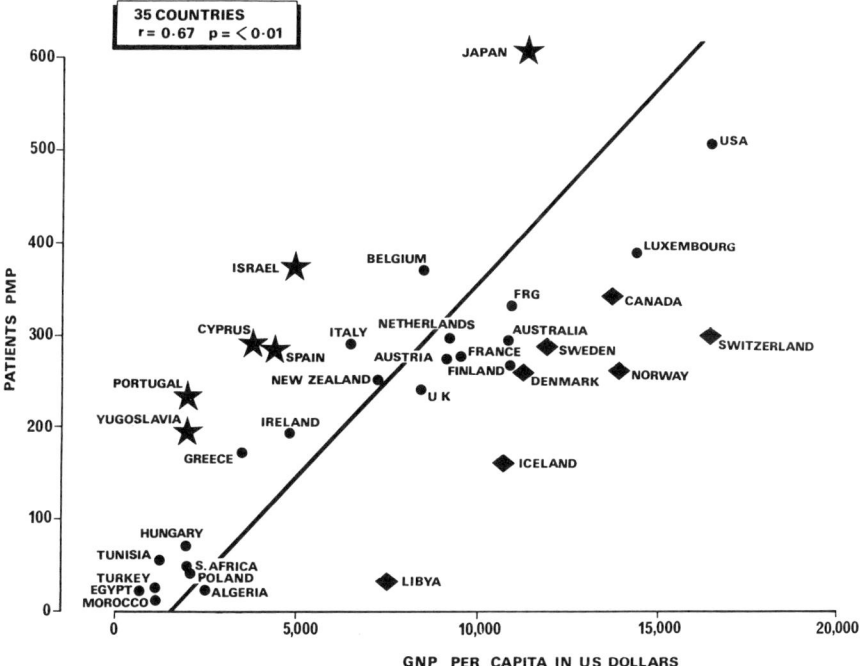

Figure 12. Relationship between total number of patients treated by dialysis and transplantation pmp and the per capita gross national project (as given in world bank atlas) in 35 countries. Reproduced from 34 with permission of the editor J.F. Maher.

222

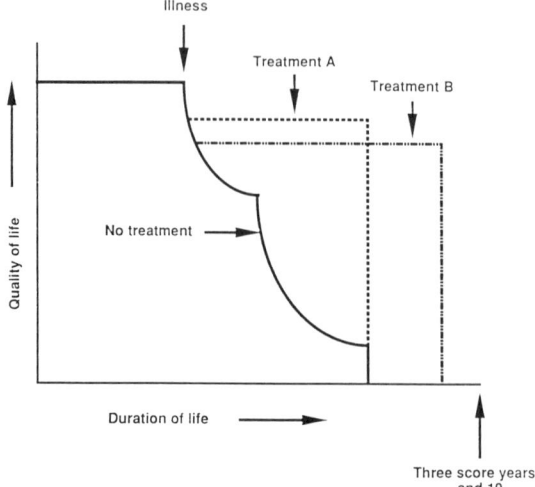

Figure 13. Graphical representation (with no numerical scale) of the duration (*x*-axis) and the quality (*y*-axis) of life, to show the impact of illness and its treatment. See text for description of lines traced by illness and treatment A and treatment B. Reproduced by permission of the Christian Medical Fellowship (U.K.).

RRT is an irrelevance. Their economies could not afford it on any scale and therefore its provision is effectively limited to a few exceptionally wealthy or favoured individuals. As far as the U.K. is concerned, we treat as many patients as would be predicted from our economic status, no more, no less.

Physicians in the U.K. who wrestle with macro allocative decisions are having to countenance the QALY (quality adjusted life year) concept [35]. This is an attempt to measure the outcome of therapies not only in terms of the survival achieved but also according to the quality of life given to the patient. Figure 13 which was suggested by the writings of Professor Alan Williams [36] illustrates the concept. Survival is measured along the *x*-axis and quality along the *y*-axis. The illness could be chronic renal failure, shortening life's span from the biblical norm 'of three score years and ten'. Treatment A represents one approach to therapy, improving quality of life over that of the untreated illness but not gaining any extra survival. Such might be achieved by the administration of erythropoeitin. Treatment B does not give such good quality but there is a clear gain in survival. Such might be achieved by diet followed by dialysis. The extra survival given by treatment B is at a quality somewhat less than a fully healthy life. If it was agreed that this decrement in quality could be quantified at, say 0.05 of the quality of healthy life, then each year of extra survival would be scored at 0.95 of a whole year. This is the QALY.

Measurements of quality are the reciprocal of valuation of illness states. The methodology of Rosser and Kind on which this is based utilizes descriptions of distress (pain) and disability (immobility) to develop a consensus through interviewing a sample of the healthy population [37].

If the costs of treatment are known then the cost per QALY for various interventions can be compared, and the comparisons used to influence macro allocative decisions. The ethic behind such an approach is essentially utilitarian, seeking the greatest good for the largest possible number of people, being prepared to discount the value of the individual patient. Proponents are liable to present it emotively by stating that expensive treatments are unethical because they take resources from the greater number of patients suffering conditions for which the remedies are less expensive.

Torrence and his group in Canada have developed another approach using the time trade-off technique as an instrument for assigning utility scales [39] and have applied it to patients on dialysis. The patient is faced with a hypothetical choice between the expected survival time, T, with his known illness and a shorter time, X, in a state of full health, subject only to normal aging processes. The interviewer adjusts X until a point of equivalence is reached. Value X/T is the utility of the health state for the individual and is scaled from 0 for death to 1.0 for perfect health. Health is defined according to the WHO as 'a state of complete physical, mental and social wellbeing and not merely the absence of disease or infirmity'.

Nephrologists in the U.K. became concerned when an attempt was made by the North West Regional Authority in association with the Centre of Health Service Economics at York University to introduce cost-QALY as a means of determining resource allocation to bids for specialty development funds. Following a debate on the 'somewhat shaky' scientific basis of the Rosser-Kind index, the Regional Medical Committee recommended that QALY methodology should not be used [35].

We do not anticipate that this rebuttal will be the last we hear of QALYs and cost QALYs. Further validation of the methodology is in hand and committees and executives faced with difficult decisions are eager for some tool of measurement to assist their deliberations.

D. *The influence of personal motives on decision making*

Do nephrologists always stand on the moral high ground in debates over the allocation of resources to their practices? Are they above being influenced by personal gain or prestige? Objective analysis and dispassionate choice is a challenge to our ethical integrity.

The method of payment for therapy and of doctors themselves has ethical impact. Fee for item of service puts a barrier between the unfunded patient and his care. The NHS was intended primarily to ensure that patients should not be denied treatment because they could not pay. Fees paid for interventions tend to act as incentives; thrice a week dialysis is selected in preference to twice a week even if the medical advantage is minimal; elderly patients are put onto dialysis even though their quality of life is deplorable; too much treatment may be prescribed [2]. Reimbursement of fees appears to be associated with the fastest inflation in medical costs and with the most litigation.

Capitation payment helps towards an equitable distribution of resources but does not provide a financial incentive to improve quality of care. The NHS uses capitation fees to fund primary care and this will be the method by which resources are distributed to purchasers (the district authorities) under the new NHS.

Salaried service, widely used to fund university posts, does not motivate towards the highest clinical workrate. It is usually associated with a system of rewards based on academic or political achievement. Since most of our renal units have hitherto been based in university or teaching hospitals this may have contributed to the inefficient use of facilities and the low numbers of patients.

Whatever method of renumeration is used, strength of professional ethic is challenged. However, it is not easy for the doctor to stand aloof from the way financial rewards cause a subtle drift in accepted clinical practice. It is only when we see obvious differences in practice, and the one variable factor which can be identified is the method of payment, that we then realise that we are all vulnerable to personal incentives. Every system houses its rogues and its saints.

The new NHS will reintroduce incentives from the marketplace. Professionals will remain salaried but their pay will be flexible and a successful institution may be able to pay higher wages and compete for the best employees. Success will depend on good management, a reputation for quality care and winning contracts to treat patients. Previously secure in our comfortable professional ethic we shall now be exposed to the winds of change blowing in from the world of competition – activity targets, critical appraisal and ruthless management.

IV. Conclusion

No health care delivery system can be judged in isolation from its historic background. The NHS has sufficed for a generation while medicine has moved on. The new NHS will, over the next few years introduce fresh constraints and incentives. Its starting point is the present situation – 43 years after the inception of the NHS, 31 years after Scribner performed repeated hemodialysis for chronic renal failure. Dialysis and transplantation have proved a severe test of whether the old style NHS could deliver a just answer. Although nephrologists have been constrained by limited resources they have seldom been restrained to prescribed numbers of patients. Decisions about who should get treatment have been perceived to have been based on clinical judgement. Operating triage, we have had a cost effective, albeit cruel system.

Will the new NHS do any better? In the future as purchasers buying packages of care, health districts will have to make explicit decisions about what they want for their populations. This may result in decisions about the level and distribution of resources receiving the sort of public attention which has accompanied the Oregon experiment in rationing healthcare [39]. Justice, if it is done, will be seen to be done: if it is not, society will share the responsibility.

Acknowledgements

I am grateful to Professor F.P. Brunner for permission to use data from the EDTA registry; and to all my friends on the EDTA registration committee for their scientific stimulus. I have quoted from data available through the South East Thames Regional Health Authority with their permission. All previously published figures are acknowledged in the Legends. I accept personal responsibility for all the views expressed in this chapter.

References

1. Wing AJ, Broyer M, Brunner FP et al. Demography of dialysis and transplantation in Europe in 1985 and 1986: trends over the previous decade. Nephrol Dial Transplant 1988; 3: 714–27.
2. Wing AJ. Renal replacement: too little or too much? In Raine AEG (ed): Advances in renal medicine. Oxford University Press: Oxford, England 1991.
3. Wing AJ. Can we meet the real need for dialysis and transplantation? Br Med J 1990; 301: 885–6.
4. Mays NB. Management and resource allocation in end-stage renal failure units: a review of current issues. Project paper number 83, King's Fund, London 1990.
5. Halper T. The misfortunes of others: end-stage renal disease- in the United Kingdom. Cambridge, University Press 1989.
6. Berlyne GM, Over 50 and uraemic = death. Nephron 1982; 31: 189–90.
7. Gokal R, McHugh M, Fryer R et al. CAPD: One year's experience in a U.K. dialysis unit. Brit Med J 1980; 281: 474–7.
8. Challah S, Wing AJ, Bauer R et al. Negative selection of patients for dialysis and transplantation in the United Kingdom. Brit Med J 1984; 288: 1119–229.
9. McGeown MG. The prevalence of advanced renal failure in Northern Ireland. Brit Med J 1990; 301: 900–3.
10. Feest TG, Mistry CD, Grimes DS et al. Incidence of advanced chronic renal failure in the United Kingdom and the need for end-stage renal replacement treatment. Brit Med J 1990; 301: 897–900.
11. Wing AJ. Medicine and the media. Brit Med J 1983; 287: 492.
12. Fassbinder W, Brunner FP, Bryngor H et al. Combined report on regular dialysis and transplantation in Europe XX. Nephrol Dial Transplant 1191 1989; 6; (suppl 1) 6–35.
13. Pincherle G. Services for patients with chronic renal failure in England and Wales. Health Trends 1977; 9: 41–44.
14. Jones NF, Mallick NP, Taube HD et al. Manpower and workload in adult renal medicine in the United Kingdom 1975–1989. J Roy Coll Physicians 1991; (in press).
15. Dalziel M, Garrett C. Intraregional variation in treating end stage renal failure. Brit Med J 1987; 294: 1382–3.
16. Smith WGJ, Cohan DR, Asscher AW. Evaluation of renal services in Wales with particular reference to the roles of subsidiary renal units: report to the Welsh office 1989. Cardiff: KRUF Institute of Renal Disease, Royal Infirmary 1989.
17. McGeown MG. Chronic renal failure in Northern Ireland, 1968–70. Lancet 1972: 1: 307–10.

226

18. Pendreight DM, Heasman MA, Howitt LF *et al*. Survey of chronic renal failure in Scotland. Lancet 1972; 1: 304–7.
19. Branch RA, Clarke GW, Cochrane AL *et al*. Incidence of uraemia and requirements for maintenance haemodialysis. Brit Med J 1971; 1: 249–54.
20. Patten J. Kidney patients. House of Commons official report (Hansard) (Dec 20) 1984; 710: col 309–10.
21. Wood IT, Mallick NP, Wing AJ. Prediction of resources needed to achieve the national target of renal failure. Br Med J 1987; 294: 1467–70.
22. H.M. Government. Working for patients: white paper on the government's proposals following its review of the NHS 1989.
23. Dorrell S. Kidney patients. House of Commons official report (Hansard) 1990; May 24: 173 cols 434–42.
24. Abel Smith B. Value for money in health services. London Heinemann 1976.
25. Mechanic D. Approaches to controlling the costs of medical care. New Eng J Med 1978; 298: 249–54.
26. Rennie D, Rettig RA, Wing AJ. Limited resources and the treatment of end-stage renal failure in Britain and United States. QJ Med 1985; 56: 34–36.
27. Cameron JS, Hogg CS, Williams DG. Treatment for renal failure in the West Midlands. Lancet 1982; 2: 1163.
28. Wing AJ. Impact of financial constraint. In Scorer CG, Wing AJ (eds): Decision making in medicine. Arnold; London 1979.
29. Calabrasi G, Bobbitt P. Tragic choices. New York: Norton 1978.
30. Halper T. Life and death in a welfare state: End stage renal disease in the United Kingdom. Millbank Mem Fund Q 1985; 63: 52–93.
31. Davison AM, Read DJ, Lewins AM. Under utilized hospital haemodialysis resources. Lancet 1984; 1: 723–5.
32. Challah S, Wing AJ, Brunner FP *et al*. Use and reuse of dialysers in Europe. In Deane, Wineman, Beamis (eds): Guide to reprocessing of haemodialysers. Martinus Nijhoff: Dordrecht 1986.
33. Taylor JE, Henderson IS, MacTier RA *et al*. Effects of withdrawing erythropoeitin. Br Med J 1991; 302: 272–3.
34. Brunner FP, Wing AJ, Dykes SR *et al*. International review of renal replacement therapy: strategies and results. In Maher JF (ed): Replacement of renal function by dialysis, 3rd edn. 1989; 697–719.
35. Wing AJ. QALYS are coming! In Quality adjusted life years: a Christian approach. Christian Medical Fellowship, London 1989.
36. Williams A. Economics of coronary artery bypass grafting. Brit Med J 1985; 291: 326–9.
37. Rosser R, Kind P. A scale of valuations of states of illness: is there a social consensus? Int J Epidemiol 1978; 7: 347–58.
38. Churchill DN, Morgan J, Torrence GW. Quality of life in end stage renal disease. Peritoneal Dial Bull 1984; 4: 20–3.
39. Klein R. On the Oregon trail; rationing healthcare. Brit Med J 1991; 302: 1–2.

18. Ethical problems in renal dialysis and transplantation: Chinese perspective

REN-ZONG QIU

This chapter consists of four sections. The first section is to provide background information on the development of renal dialysis and transplantation in the Peoples Republic of China (PRC). In the second and third sections I discuss the macro-allocation and micro-allocation problems in the application of renal dialysis and transplantation in China, respectively. Other ethical problems are addressed in the fourth section.

I. Renal dialysis and transplantation in China

Renal dialysis and transplantation were first introduced into China in the 1950s and 1960s respectively. Since the middle of the 1950s, dialysis for patients with acute renal failure (ARF) has been developed. In the period 1955–1982, 478 (21.9%) of 2,182 cases of ARF all over the country, were treated with dialysis. In the period 1982–1987, out of 1,918 cases of ARF, 1,716 (91.8%) were treated with hemodialysis, and 157 (8.2%) with peritoneal dialysis. In some clinics CAVH or AVHDF has been developed recently [15].

The annual incidence of chronic end-stage renal diseases is about 10/100,000, that is 110,000 patients per year. At the end of 1987, there were 762 artificial kidneys used in 305 clinics. The number of patients who have been treated with dialysis totals 11,591, a 27.5% increase compared to 1986. The incidence of end-stage renal diseases in Japan seems to be similar to China, but according to the statistics of 1985 there were 28,715 artificial kidneys and the number of patients dialyzed totalled 66,310 [15].

The application of kidney transplantation began in the 1960s, but was only given publicity in 1974. In the 1970s a nation-wide upsurge of organ transplantation was set off, including kidney, liver, heart and lung transplantation, but it turned to be at low ebb because of the shortage of donated organs and unacceptance of the 'brain death' concept in China [13]. According to statistics, up to December 1989 there were 122 clinics in which kidney transplantation had been developed. In 1989, kidney transplantation was performed on 1,049 patients in 42 clinics [12]. In a report of the First National Conference on

227

C. M. Kjellstrand and J. B. Dossetor (eds): Ethical Problems in Dialysis and Transplantation, 227–235.
© 1992 *Kluwer Academic Publishers. Printed in the Netherlands.*

Organ Transplantation it was disclosed that cadaver kidney transplantation has been performed on 2,435 cases, with 2,707 cadaver kidneys to the end of 1987. In some hospitals the one year survival rate of the transplanted kidneys reached about 80%–90% [12] compared to 56.25% in 1985 [14]. Even in a provincial grade hospital the 1 year survival rate reached 56.14% and over the 5 year survival 32.26% during 1978–1988 [7].

Professor Qiu Fazu, Director of Institute of Organ Transplantation in Wuhan, identified the following problems facing Chinese doctors in organ transplantation.

1. The most urgent problem which has to be solved is the difficulty of organ procurement which causes a serious shortage of organs and no guarantee of quality. This in turn is associated with the un-acceptability of 'brain death' concept.
2. Setting up an organization to co-ordinate the procurement, preservation and distribution of organs all over the country.
3. Heart and liver transplantation has been suspended in recent years and the units performing kidney transplantation have decreased since 1982.
4. Searching for an efficient and cheaper immunosuppressant [8].

II. The problem of macro-allocation in renal dialysis and transplantation

I think the problem of justice and injustice in kidney dialysis and transplantation consists mainly of problems of macro-allocation and micro-allocation. Dr. Tom Beauchamp discusses micro-allocation by first asking whether we are justified as a society in not allocating the resources necessary to treat dialysis patients, and examines micro-allocation by asking whether we are justified in withholding dialysis in particular cases [1]. Put in a positive way, the first question to be asked is what resources can be justifiably allocated to deliver renal dialysis and/or transplantation to patients, and the second question is to ask what kind of criteria, medical as well as social, is justifiably prescribed for choosing which patients to treat with dialysis or transplantation.

The preferred policy in China is that renal dialysis or transplantation not be given priority in the agenda of health care delivery. It means that the resources which are allocated to them are lower than those given to cancer or cardiovascular/cerebro-vascular diseases.

This policy might be justified as follows:

(1) Kidney diseases together with reproductive diseases occupy eighth place in the list of the first ten main killers in some cities, and tenth in that of some counties (Table 1):

Table 1. Specific mortality of the first ten main diseases in some cities and counties (1987) [16]

(1) Cities

Cause of death	Specific mortality (1/100,000)	Percentage (%) in total deaths
1. Malignant tumours	131.99	21.61
2. Cerebrovascular diseases	125.89	20.61
3. Heart diseases	92.84	15.20
4. Respiratory diseases	91.83	15.08
5. Injuries and poisonings	46.46	7.61
6. Digestive diseases	27.42	4.49
7. Newborn diseases	955.41 (1/100,000 live births)	1.99
8. Urological & reproductive diseases	10.06	1.65
9. Pulmonary tuberculosis	9.83	1.61
10. Endocrinous, nutritional & metabolic diseases	9.01	1.47
Subtotal		91.32

(2) Counties

Cause of death	Specific mortality (1/100,000)	Percentage (%) in total deaths
1. Respiratory diseases	143.06	20.83
2. Cerebrovascular diseases	101.87	14.83
3. Malignant tumours	97.45	13.19
4. Heart diseases	89.74	13.07
5. Injuries & poisonings	70.53	10.27
6. Digestive diseases	34.53	5.03
7. Pulmonary tuberculosis	20.22	2.94
8. Newborn diseases	975.05 (1/100,000 live births)	2.30
9. Infectious diseases (Except pulmonary tuberculosis)	14.30	2.09
10. Urological & reproductive diseases	8.09	1.18
Subtotal		86.73

If we had unlimited resources, we would have dealt with all these diseases at the same time, regardless of expense, but we have not had, and perhaps never will have, such resources, in a developing country such as China. In the period 1980–1986, the sum of funds allocated to health care, and its percentage in national expenditure was as follows (Table 2):

We cannot do everything with limited resources. It might be argued that it is not appropriate to allocate such limited funding to health care services, but this is another problem. For instance, in a Colloqium on Reform and Development of Health Care, held in Beijing, November 16–18, 1988, I argued that it is unethical to allocate only 3% of national expenditure to health care or education. Even though the resources allocated to health care are appropriate, they are always limited. We

Table II. Sum of funds for health care and its percentage in national expenditure (1980–1986) [16]

Year	Sum of funds for health care (billion yuan)	Percentage in national expenditure (%)
1980	3.01652	2.49
1981	3.274	2.94
1982	3.766	3.27
1983	4.195	3.25
1984	4.816	3.11
1985	5.481	2.97
1986	6.428	2.79

have to set an order of priority. As only the eighth or tenth of the top killers, renal diseases cannot enjoy the primary concern in the current condition. One Chinese saying states:

If you want to do something, you have to forget about doing something else.

(2) Within the limited resources allocated to the delivery of medical services for renal disease, the emphasis should be put on prevention, early treatment, treatment of pre-end-stage renal diseases, and non-dialysis treatment. An ancient Chinese physician argued that:

The sage does not treat those who have already been ill, but those who have not yet been ill [4].

A Chinese physician in medieval times named Zhu Zhenheng [17] said:

It is better to promote health earlier than to treat disease and save the life later. For it is usually in vain to resort to medicine when the disease has already invaded the body. Therefore, the maxim of doctors is not to treat those who have already fallen ill. To treat those who have not fallen ill, we have to understand the truth of preserving life. If we think of all possible troubles and take adequate preventive measures, nothing has to be worried about. This is what is meant by not treating those who have already fallen ill, but those who have not.

It may be charged with evasion of responsibility to say not to treat those who have already fallen ill, but those who have not. However, it is right to put emphasis on prevention and early treatment. I agree with Dr. Louanne Kennedy [5] who says that today's ethos, as well as in the current framework of health care system of many countries, the major concern is preventing deaths rather than promoting health.

(3) Up to now, kidney dialysis or transplantation is still an experimental and expensive treatment, at least in our country. As an experimental treatment we have

to limit it to use within a few centers, with medically and ethically competent physicians and researchers. Dr. Arthur Caplan [2] is right when he says:

> Medical ethicists misunderstood the normative problem involving renal dialysis. The real issue during the late 1960's and early 1970's was not 'who should suvive?' or 'who gets the machine?', but rather, when should a new technology be treated as a therapy available to all, rather than as an experiment available only to a very select few?

Dialysis machines and transplantation are too expensive to be afforded by the public health care services of which the only beneficiaries are workers and professionals in state-owned factories or institutions, and many patients will never enjoy the benefits. In China, the cost of hemodialysis is about 350 yuan (about $70.00 U.S.) per treatment and 40,000 yuan (about 8,000.00 U.S.) per year, and the cost of kidney transplantation from a cadaver is about 20,000 yuan (about $4,000.00 U.S.), mainly for the cost of imported cyclosporin A. But the funds for public health care services is only about 50 yuan (about $10.00 U.S.) per person, per year, in Peking Union Hospital. There are now 2,400 members of this hospital, so the funds for public health services for members are about 120,000 yuan (about $24,000.00 U.S.) per year. This means that the total funds can only support the cost of hemodialysis for 3 persons per year, or the cost of kidney transplantation for 6 persons per year. Those who have no access to public health services have maybe an average salary of about 200 yuan (about $50.00 U.S.) per person, per month. Perhaps only the few rich who have emerged since the new economic policy, can afford the costs.

III. The problem of micro-allocation in renal dialysis and transplantation

Limited resources have made the micro-allocation problem more acute. If the statistics of the incidence of end-stage renal diseases, which show a figure of 10/100,000 per year, are correct, the number of new patients with this disease each year would be 110,000, given that China's population is now 1.1 billion. Unfortunately, there are only 762 artificial dialysis machines and at the end of 1988 only 11,591 patients had been dialyzed, so only a few patients with end-stage renal diseases are given access to hemodialysis.

Now what are the medical and social criteria available for choosing patients for renal dialysis and transplantation? There are some conventions, but no written guidelines or regulations.

Apart from indications and contraindications, the major concern is on preventing death or improving the quality of life after treatment. A male patient in his 40's has now survived for 11 years since his renal transplantation in Peking Union Hospital, and has done very well in his position as a researcher of scientific information.

As Dr. C.M. Kjellstrand pointed out [6], there is a difference between dialysis and transplantation. The former is a life-saving measure, and the latter, if successful, will improve the quality of life considerably. Therefore in many clinics, patients who are chosen for dialysis are also the candidates for renal transplantation.

There is no age barrier for dialysis, but the elderly appear to be denied access to renal transplantation. There is no sex barrier for dialysis and transplantation, although the data show that the percentage of male patients undergoing renal transplantation is much higher than that of female patients (Table 3).

Table III. Age and sex difference in 79 cases of renal transplantation from cadavers (August 1978– March 1988) [7]

Age	%	Sex	No. of Patients	%
19 – 31	59.49	Male	59	74.7
32 – 45	31.64	Female	20	25.3
46 – 49	8.87			

What about the social criteria for choosing patients? In contrast with the American and other Western countries where people are accustomed to right-language, contemporary Chinese get used to benefit or profit-language. This is not the Confucian tradition. At the beginning of the third century B.C. when King Hui of Liang first met Mencius, one of the Great Confucianists, he asked him: 'Will you bring some profits to my country coming from thousands of miles away?' Mencius answered: 'Why must Your Majesty use the term profit? What I have to offer is nothing but humanity and righteousness' ([13] p. 60).

But now, Chinese are used to arguing about what ought to be done in terms of how much benefit (in Chinese benefit, profit and utility are expressed by the same character ('li'), will be obtained from it. Benefit to whom? To the society at large, to the community or the working unit, or to individuals and their families? In the language of contemporary Chinese, the benefit is usually classified into economic and social benefit. For instance, if we save the life of a skilful worker or of a bright and capable engineer, we can estimate the economic benefit to his/her family and working unit. If the patient is of high ranking cadre or a distinguished professor, to save his/her life would have other benefits than economic ones, including political or moral implications, called social benefits. Although I have argued that there is something more important than economic and social benefit, there is something we have to do even if there are no clear benefits from doing it [9]. But my voice is no more than a noise against the overwhelming benefit-language background. An even greater problem is how to quantify various kinds of benefits and how to calculate them, and then to agree on who should do the calculations.

Anyway, there are some valuable considerations in this benefit language that might be taken into practical account in all countries. Among the patients who will have a considerably improved quality of life after treatment are those who have made contributions and/or will probably make potential contributions to society and/or mankind. These are the patients who should be given priority access to treatment. In China it is considered probable that persons in higher rank cadres or on the higher grade on the wage scale have made or will make more contributions. But that is not necessarily the case. We should have set criteria for assessing the contributions a person has made or will make, through a democratic mechanism, and set up ethical committees in hospitals to apply these criteria to particular cases.

I do not think that either choosing patients for transplantation by first come, first serve, or by lottery, is a good idea. First come, first serve, may be used as a secondary principle, if other conditions are the same for two patients. Choosing by lottery is only a method of shirking responsibility and dodging difficulties, and leaving the choices to God.

There is a financial barrier for patients. In state-owned institutions the funds for public health care are fixed and allocated by central or local government, but not in state-owned enterprises. The funds for labour insurance for example, in a factory, depend on its performance, and are provided by the factory itself. Funds in a well-managed factory are much higher than those in a poorly managed factory. Even if a patient meets all criteria, medical as well as social, access to dialysis or transplantation is denied because the cost is much beyond what can be afforded by the factory to which he or she is affiliated.

Is this unjust to those patients who are barred from dialysis or transplantation for financial reasons or shortage of machines or organs? Yes, in the sense that their condition dictates treatment with dialysis or transplantation, but under the present conditions we cannot avoid all unfortunate events, and sometimes we have to choose the lesser of two evils.

What can be done for patients who are not given access to dialysis or transplantation. The quite efficient techniques of peritoneal dialysis and enema with traditional medicine have been developed in recent years in China. We should put more stress on developing these treatments even without sensational news value.

IV. Cultural barriers to renal dialysis and transplantation

China is now a society with changing values. I have talked about bioethics in the Peoples Republic of China with the title of 'Morality in Flux' [1]. Some contemporary Chinese are more westernized and have no trouble in accepting any modern technology. Some are more traditional, modern technology is alien to them. We have reported a case in which a traditional family refused to accept even a male baby with AIDS [10].

In Chinese culture, what is valued is the natural (for Taoists) or meaningful (for Confucianists) life. For Confucianists what is valued is not the human life itself, but to live in an ideal way. The great historian Sima Qian (145–90 B.C.) said that every person has to die, somebody's death is as heavy as the Tai Mountains, somebody's death is as light as the feather of a wild goose. Confucius once said:

A man of humanity will never seek to live at the expense of injuring humanity. He would rather sacrifice his life in order to realize humanity ([3], p. 43).

In other words, what is valued is the meaningful and not meaningless life. The meaning of life for Confucianists is to follow Confucian ethical principles which teach people to be human – worthy members of the universal family.

Moreover, for Confucianists, to live or die is not something which can be controlled by human beings. Confucius said:

Life and death are the chance of Heaven, wealth and honor depend on Heaven ([3] p. 39).

The only thing we can control is what we ought to do, so the logical consequence is to let nature take its course on the matter of life and death.

One school of Taoism emphasizes the preserving of life by means of breathing, exercise, diet, sex and medicine. What they want to preserve is a natural existence, in which will be maintained a harmony or balance of Yin and Yang within the human body, and between the body and the universe. It implies the principle of 'non-action' ('wu wei'), which does not mean 'do nothing', but rather, do nothing unnatural or beyond nature.

But the question, what is natural life and what is unnatural life, remain to be reidentified and re-interpreted in the new circumstances. It seems that the prolonging of dying of a terminally ill patient can be identified as an unnatural life, but how about the life after dialysis and transplantation? It might be identified as an unnatural life if we consider another principle – filial piety in Chinese tradition. In one of the Confucian classics entitled *Book of Filial Piety* it was said that hair and skin, which are inherited from parents, should not be damaged. According to this principle, dissecting of the human body, and all major operations including the donation of organs, have to be prohibited, and only non-invasive treatment developed in Traditional Chinese Medicine. Renal dialysis and transplantation damage not only hair and skin, but also pierce a hole through the body, or open to cavity to remove an original organ which comes from the parents, and replace it with another one which comes from an alien. It would definitely violate the principle of filial piety if the traditional values are insisted upon. Thus, life after dialysis or transplantation might be regarded as an unnatural existence. This may explain why some Chinese who insist on traditional values, reject dialysis and transplantation, even when in a critical condition, and the quality of life would be improved with treatment.

References

1. Beauchamp T. Can we stop or withhold dialysis?, in Schreiner GE (ed): Proceedings of the First Conference, Controversies in Nephrology. Washington, DC. 1979; pp. 18–19.
2. Caplan AL. Applying morality to advances in biomedicine: can and should this be done?, in Bondeson WB *et al.* (eds): New knowledge in the biomedical sciences: Some moral implications of its acquisition, possession, and use. D. Reidel Dordrecht 1982; pp. 155–168.
3. Chan WT. A source book in Chinese philosophy. Princeton University Press: New Jersey, Princeton 1963.
4. The Interior Classics of Yellow Emperor: Plain Iniquities. People Health Press 1963; p. 14.
5. Kennedy L. Choices posed by alternative treatment modalities for end-stage renal disease. J Health Polit Policy Law 1980; 5 (2): 368–374.
6. Kjellstrand CM. Giving life, giving death, Ethical problems with high technology medicine. Ph.D. Thesis, Karolinska Institute, Stockholm 1988 and Acta Medica Scandinavica Suppl 1988; Suppl 725.
7. Li JQ *et al.* Experience on 90 cases/times kidney transplantation from cadavers. Chinese J Org Transpl 1990; 11 (2): 9–1.
8. Qiu FZ. Congratulations on the founding of the Chinese society of organ transplantation and best wishes to its 1st congress. Chi J Org Transpl 1988; 9 (3): 97.
9. Qiu RZ. The interaction between science-technology and culture. Newsletter of Dialectics of Nature 1988; (3), July.
10. Qiu RZ. AID confronts the law in China. Hastings Center Report 1989; 19 (6): 3–4.
11. Qiu RZ. Morality in flux: bioethics in PRC. J of Kennedy Inst of Ethics (In print)
12. Register Office of Organ Transplantation. A 1989 statistics of kidney transplantation in China. Chi J Org Transpl 1990; 11 (2): 86.
13. Xia SS. Developing new styles of operation to raise the level of 1990's organ transplantation. Chi J Org Transpl 1990; 11 (1): 1–2.
14. Xie T *et al.* Experience on 107 cases of organ transplantation. Chi J Org Transpl 1985; 6 (3): 113.
15. Xie T. The blood purification of the country is going forward. Chi J Org Transpl 1989; 6 (3): 113.
16. The Year Book of Health Care. People Health Press, Beijing, 1988; pp. 558–563.
17. Zhu ZH. On not treating those who have fallen ill, but those who have not, in Selections of ancient medical texts. Shanghai Science-Technology Press 1980; p. 146.
18. Zhou XX. A report on the first national conference on organ transplantation of Chinese Medical Association. Chi J Org Transpl 1989; 10 (1): 42–43.

Developments in Nephrology

Developments in Nephrology

Kluwer Academic Publishers – Dordrecht / Boston / London